unsung love song

unsung love song

—

laurence dillon

First published 2020

by Zuleika Books & Publishing

Thomas House, 84 Eccleston Square
London, SW1V 1PX

British Library Cataloguing in Publication Data

A catalogue record for this book is
available from the British Library

ISBN: 978-1-9161977-3-2

Designed by Euan Monaghan
Printed in England

WARNING

contains material that may be
considered disturbing and offensive

Prologue

I was sick the day it all began. I vomited several times – maybe it was coincidence, or perhaps my body was telling me that something was wrong. I went into work as normal and started my night shift at the local hospital, as a radiographer – someone has to do it.

The hospital was a self-contained world with its unique rhythms and rituals, its own peculiar protocols. I belonged. I liked my job and enjoyed feeling that I was part of something bigger than me. I was proud to be involved with an important and worthwhile endeavour. I "believed" in the NHS.

It was the week before Christmas and the evening was busy with a constant stream of patients arriving, but it slowed down after midnight. The X-ray department could be a hectic place during the day, but in the small hours it often became quiet and still: the gentle hum of equipment could be heard now that the general day-time commotion wasn't drowning it out.

I was the only member of staff on duty in X-ray that night. There was a bell that was rung every time a patient was sent for X-ray from Accident & Emergency. It hadn't sounded for a while. I also carried a bleeper for any urgent in-patient X-rays, but that was silent as well.

In the lull, I made myself a cup of tea and sat in the staff room on my own, glad that it was peaceful now.

Later, I went to the toilet. Sitting on the seat, I pulled gently at the toilet-roll on the wall. I absentmindedly doubled up two squares together and reached down between my legs. What? That's really odd! One of my balls was enormous, the right one. A stream of questions crowded urgently into my consciousness, my mind frantically trying to answer them. What's going on? I have no idea. How did this happen? I don't know. Was this new? Yes. Finally, a question I could answer. Yes, it was new – I hadn't noticed it before; it seemed to me that it must have happened suddenly. I cupped them both in my hand. Yes, the right one was definitely twice the size of the left one. There was no discomfort; in fact, it felt quite numb.

I made an effort to be rational and methodically considered the possibilities, reminding myself that I shouldn't jump to conclusions about testicular cancer. "It's not the likeliest cause," I told myself, whilst also thinking– "please don't let it be *that*!"

It was most probably an infection, I reasoned, whilst pondering the matter back in the staff room. The bell rang, indicating a patient, and I put the matter out of my mind whilst I concentrated on my professional role. Once the patient had been returned to the A&E department, I visited the toilet again for another look. Yes, it was still the same. No, it hadn't shrunk back to its customary size. I had hoped that it might have been some sort of late-night hallucination, but it wasn't. The ball was hard and swollen; I could flick it with my finger and not feel anything much. I did it four or five times. Still nothing. Something was definitely not right here.

I thought for a moment and had an idea. Making myself presentable, I walked along the empty corridor to the porter's room. There were two of them there, sitting with their feet resting upon a scuffed tabletop, a radio playing in the background. I asked one of them if he would let me into the Urology department (it was closed at night), saying I needed to get something that I'd left there. He nodded and got up, walking with me to the nearby department and unlocked the door, waiting outside as I nipped in to achieve my secret objective. I pressed a switch near the door and the strip-lighting flickered above me. Quickly, I walked towards the display racks with all the free leaflets – the leaflets that explain different diagnoses, answer questions, outline symptoms, red flags and alarm bells. Within a minute I had accomplished my mission, tucking the leaflets into my pockets discreetly. I switched the lights off, thanked the porter, told myself that the deception had been in a good cause.

Once back in my own department I carefully read the information leaflets – they described testicular hydroceles, torsions…and cancer. I went through them over and over. There were a few things that could cause a swollen testicle; that was reassuring.

When the day staff came on in the morning and my shift was over, I acted as normal, and went home as usual. This time though, I phoned my local health centre and made an appointment to see a GP before falling into bed.

Two days later I saw a locum doctor who prescribed a course of antibiotics, then muttered something about having the testicle removed if they didn't have any effect. That sort of remark might have freaked out many guys, but I had read the leaflets and felt sure it was going to be alright. Anyway, I wasn't the sort of chap who let self-indulgent feelings get the better of him, was I? No, not me. Little did I know that a tiny little black-hole, smaller than a pinhead, was being born in a galaxy far away – deep inside me.

I was confident that the matter would soon be concluded and quickly forgotten about. I mentioned my big ball to a couple of friends who were nurses, and they reckoned it was very likely a hydrocele – a collection of fluid. But a week later, it was still enormous, which wasn't encouraging. That indicated that the antibiotics hadn't worked – and that it therefore probably wasn't an infection.

As December approached its end, my swollen ball was still the same size. I enjoyed the customary Christmas celebrations all the same, the only drawback being that I was going to be working New Year's Eve – a particularly demanding shift. New Year's Eve in A&E is always a slightly crazy experience.

Once I'd finished the course of antibiotics, I went back to see my GP. He asked me a few questions – did I feel any pain? No, I didn't. Had the testicle altered over the last week? No, it hadn't. After hearing my answers, and doing a brief examination, he sent me for further investigation at the local hospital – the same one I worked in. I had to get someone to cover my shift. Later that day, instead of being a member of staff, I sat on a bed in a ward as a patient, listening to a junior doctor explaining to me that I may have a sexually trans-mitted disease (STD) such as chlamydia or gonorrhoea – both of which were associated with swollen testicles. An ultrasound scan was requested, and I was sent home. An STD sounded like quite a desirable diagnosis to me, actually; certainly, when compared with cancer.

A few days afterwards I lay on a couch in a little room in the radiology department. I was given a piece of blue tissue-paper to hold my penis up against my body, so that it wouldn't get in the way. The transducer probe was pressed firmly against my testicles as the consultant radiologist looked at the screen and moved the probe to get the best pictures. It was strange to be a patient in my own department, and here I was having my balls prod-ded by a chap I worked with.

He didn't say anything as he did the scan, and I knew better than to ask any questions – he'd have to review the images before making his report. I wasn't going to be one of those staff-members who are an awkward patient;

I was just going to let people get on with their jobs. I'd find out soon enough. And I did – he broke it to me right there and then, as soon as I'd wiped the gel off my balls with the piece of blue tissue paper and pulled my underpants and trousers up.

It was malignancy – cancer. He said that he would report the images urgently and arrange for the surgeon to see me. I thanked him, and vaguely sensed a slight tremor emanate from the undiscovered black hole inside me. Apart from that, I didn't feel much. 'Phlegmatic' could have been my middle name. Half an hour later I was telling my manager that I might be taking a little time off work, as it looked like I might have a touch of cancer. You know, like having a bit of a cold or something. He didn't say much, but I was officially put on sick leave.

The consultant surgeon saw me for the first time later that day in a room behind a wide wooden door with a big frosted window. He sat behind a desk, with some hospital notes in front of him. It was an old desk, well-made, but the varnish had peeled off over the years. One of his team was there too, whilst a Macmillan nurse stood poised at the back, ready to step forward if things got a bit emotional. Her head was angled slightly; her face bore an expression of empathy which contrasted with the detached manner of the doctor. Probably some people don't react too well to hearing bad news. Well, I was going to be just fine actually. I felt that distant stirring within me again but refused to pay it any attention.

The consultant spoke quickly. I took in the information calmly. He informed me that I had been diagnosed with a type of malignancy called teratoma. I had just been told I had cancer, but I might just as well have been told that I had dandruff. There was no outward reaction from me – the doctor delivered the news matter-of-factly and I accepted it politely. I felt a sinking feeling in my abdomen but obeyed the mantra that echoed in my head – no matter what happens, act with *dignity*. Things were turning out exactly as I had hoped they wouldn't, but I had drawn up an action plan that I intended to follow. *Dignity*, I thought to myself. There are plenty of people worse off than you, just you remember that! My personal black hole got a little bit bigger again, and I didn't notice it at all.

But if one piece of bad news wasn't enough, there was an unexpected complication – the ultrasound scan had indicated a probable teratoma in my left testicle too. The surgeon told me that he thought it best to deal with one issue at a time and decided to operate on my swollen testicle first. I was booked in for an orchidectomy – removal of testicle. He told me what would happen in the operation: that he would make an incision in my lower abdomen and pull the testicle up along the inguinal canal and out from the incision. My spermatic cord would be clamped, then snipped, and it's done.

Finally, he asked me if I'd like a prosthetic testicle inserted after the diseased one had been removed, I shrugged my shoulders and said yes. I visited my department later to look at one of the medical textbooks kept on a shelf there and found out more about teratoma: how it is a germ cell tumour that arises in cells which produce eggs or sperm. Women can get teratoma too, it affects their ovaries.

I travelled home on the bus, blankly looking at the grey winter day through a rain-splattered window. Back home, I slumped down on the sofa and rang my mother. I told her the news and she started crying. I reassured her that everything was going to be okay. She was a doctor, so knew that I was probably not in any great mortal danger, but she was also my mum. It made me feel uncomfortable to know that I had caused her to be upset.

I called some friends and met them in a pub later that evening, determined to get very drunk. After a couple of beers, I realised that alcohol wasn't going to have any effect on me at all, so we went for something to eat instead. It was good to spend time talking about sport, music, films – any subject but the unfortunate bombshell that had crashed into my life. When any of them asked me how I felt about the news, I told them that I was fine. After all, as far as I knew, I *was* fine. I certainly wasn't going to indulge in any emotional outbursts or displays of weakness. In actual fact, I didn't really know how I felt. Unrealised by me at the time, I had shut down my emotions and was allowing an autopilot to guide me.

8

At home, I looked at the leaflet about testicular cancer that I'd got a fortnight before and read through it again. In percentage terms, the survival rate for those with a testicular cancer diagnosis is in the nineties, so I wasn't unduly worried. It carried on to say that boys with a history of undescended testes had a higher incidence of developing testicular cancer in adult life. That struck a chord with me – I had undergone an operation for un-descended testicles when I was ten, or maybe eleven. My brother had told other boys at school about this, which resulted in me being baited about having had my balls amputated. I recalled the mockery with a cold shiver.

Two mornings later I was admitted onto one of the surgical wards; the first time I'd been an in-patient since I was a boy. Back then I'd had my balls fixed in place, this time I was going to have one of them removed. The pre-surgery checks were done. Eventually, after a lot of waiting about, I was wheeled down to theatre. It's weird being pushed along a corridor where people you pass keep recognising you, but I just smiled at them or offered a cheery greeting if they looked questioningly at me. I knew the anaesthetist too and chatted to him as he prepared to put me under, all the while just wanting to be sent to sleep and to have it all over with. A mask was placed over my face, my body felt tense and rigid, my heart was thumping hard. I heard a voice scream in my head – "Please just knock me out!" It was my voice, and no-one could hear it except me.

Once the anaesthetic had taken full effect, I'd be wheeled through a set of doors into the theatre. I'd be transferred onto the operating table; there'd be a couple of surgeons, a scrub nurse, a runner (a nurse who charts equipment use and helps the scrub nurse), an ODA (operating department assistant), and maybe one or two more people there. After about an hour and a half, I'd be put on a trolley again and sent back to the ward.

I was really groggy when I woke up in bed. Everything had gone well, apparently, but I felt awful. My lower abdomen was very sore, and I felt nauseous. One of the nurses offered me morphine but I said I'd be okay – I wasn't going to trouble anyone; I was going to be a model patient. A friend who was a nurse visited me later and said I should have grabbed the chance of morphine, as it was really good stuff. My parents came to see me just after the operation, but I wasn't at my best then.

I was touched when friends came to visit me later; even just a quick "hello" is really good for a patient's morale. A few people popped in from my department to see how I was, and jokingly told me to stop malingering and get back to work as soon as possible.

A couple of days later I was sent home and felt a lot better by then. My groin was bruised, swollen, and tender. I was given a surgical harness to wear: I called it my "ball bag". The swelling went down after a few days, but it seemed that I had picked up an infection as red spots appeared on the head of my penis – a real case of spotted dick. A strong dose of antibiotics sorted that out. I didn't do much during those first days after surgery; read books, listened to music, watched the occasional film on television.

After a week or so I was back at the surgical clinic again. The consultant said that a decision had to be taken concerning my remaining testicle. In view of the ultrasound report, it was probably going to have to be removed as well. The surgeon carried on talking, breezing over the subject easily. I felt that sinking feeling again, but concentrated on playing my role of philosophical stoic, and I think I pulled it off rather well actually. I'd spoken with my mother on the 'phone about the forthcoming operation. She had made it clear that the wisest course of action was to remove the second ball too. Safety first – don't take any risks. This seemed sensible and logical, but I had to make more of an effort to put on the "yeah-I'm-really-fine-with-it" act now that it had begun to become clear to me that I was going to be neutered.

I got the bus home, looking out of the window but not really seeing anything, reminding myself to keep my dignity. I was not going to be a whiner. Everything was going to be fine. *Dignity*, I thought to myself. Just keep it together.

The Oncology team arranged for me to have a CT scan at the regional cancer hospital to make sure that the malignancy had not spread to anywhere else in my body.

In the waiting room I sat opposite a young woman in her twenties who was accompanied by her mother. The woman wore a scarf over her head; she had no hair. I told myself how fortunate I was to only be a day-tripper to the cancer theme park. I repeated this to myself once the CT report came through, stating that the cancer had not spread.

In late January, I received an appointment for the Fertility Laboratory at the maternity hospital so that I could bank some sperm before it was too late. I had never been a father; maybe I could still be one someday? A chatty lady explained the legal aspects of sperm storage. I didn't really take in much of what she said but signed the forms that she put in front of me. Then she gave me a bottle, led me along the corridor, and showed me through a door which she then closed behind me.

Suddenly I was standing alone in a room containing a chair, an examination bed, and bedside cabinet. The last thing I felt like doing was the very thing I was here to do. Unscrewing the lid of the little empty bottle that I'd been given, I read the label; it already had my name upon it, and a number. Oh dear!

Absentmindedly, I opened the drawer of the cabinet. Ah, the lady hadn't told me that there would be magazines to help things along. Glossy, quite new, not dog-eared or damaged – yes, I could work with those. I concentrated, flicking through pages of girls until I found the one I liked best. Come on, I thought, pull yourself together – you can do this. You're a guy – it's in your job description for goodness sake.

I managed it eventually and returned to reception with the bottle – lid securely in place. I was shown through to a laboratory where I was invited to look through a microscope at a few lonely sperm wandering around. The lady explained that I had produced a very small quantity of sperm, but this didn't mean that I was completely infertile. She told me that, in view of my low sperm count, I would need to attend quite a few times to produce a viable amount. An appointment was made for my next visit.

It was much easier the second time around. Most guys produce enough sperm after one or two visits, but I needed quite a few more – they could have issued me with a season-ticket.

By now it was February, and for a few surreal weeks I made several visits to that little room to make further deposits. I only had one abnormal testicle then; it was probably for the chop soon enough, and it wasn't producing much. I was still on sick-leave and would catch a train into Manchester, then walk along Oxford Road if it was a nice day or catch a bus if it was raining. Once I jumped into a taxi because I was late for my appointment.

The magazines seemed to change regularly; it was as if there was some sort of soft-core library in operation. On one visit they all featured ladies with enormous plastic breasts, making it rather difficult – that's not really my thing. I had to close my eyes and use my imagination to get the job done. The next time I had an appointment there I stopped off beforehand at a newsagent to ensure classier material for myself and my fellow wankers. I checked the place was empty before scooping a broad selection off the top shelf and going to the counter. A girl appeared out of nowhere and stood beside me whilst we waited for the shopkeeper to stop messing about with the cigarettes. I blushed as she looked at me and my pile of purchases with obvious contempt. I thought better of informing her that it was all for a good cause. She didn't look like she'd see the funny side.

All the while I was making these visits that had become bizarrely normal, the prosthetic testicle was causing a problem. It had become infected and sore and was eroding through my scrotum. When the consultant surgeon saw it, he said that it would be removed along with the remaining diseased one – but that didn't turn out to be necessary. One evening at the end of February I had quite a bit of lower abdominal discomfort and when I dropped my trousers, the silicon prosthesis bounced upon the floor and the pain was relieved instantly. There was a hole in my scrotum, an exit wound which healed up after a couple of weeks. I still have the artificial ball at home somewhere – a strange souvenir.

Another ultrasound scan was done in early March on my remaining testicle; the report indicated teratoma once more. I asked the surgeon if it might be possible to conduct a biopsy to confirm the diagnosis; he stated that it was not. I had hoped that it might be possible to avoid losing both balls as this was going to have a greater impact than just losing one. I went to the hospital's medical library and found a surgery textbook which explained that testicular biopsies presented a risk of opening new pathways for malignancy to spread within the patient's body. I told myself that being castrated was better than being dead, so that was all that there was to it. I didn't feel anything really. I wasn't going to allow myself to feel anything.

It seemed more straight-forward the second time around. Once again, I found myself being wheeled down the corridor; once again I behaved as cheerfully as possible to any colleagues that passed. The anaesthetist informed me that he was going to use an alternative as they'd had to give me enough anaesthetic before the first orchidectomy to knock out an elephant. He gave me an injection this time – I only heard the screams in my head for a short while before it took effect. I woke up back in the ward, with my parents at the bedside. I felt much better than I had the first time; the anaesthetic was perhaps more agreeable to me. I was discharged after a couple of days with a temporary limp and no balls, ready to get on with my life.

I had accepted my lot, or at least was trying very hard to, but what made it rather more difficult was an unforeseen development that was going to make it all considerably more awkward for me psychologically.

A week after the operation, the histopathology report came back. I had been through this before with the first operation so I reckoned that I knew the script – the surgeon would sit there and drily confirm that the report found a teratoma malignancy. Only this time, there was a little surprise. The consultant explained that the histopathology report stated that there had been no malignancy present in my left testicle. There had been a benign abnormality – an epidermoid cyst. Oh! This would have been fantastic news if my ball had not already been removed, but as he spoke, I processed what he was telling me. Through the jargon and the words, the conclusion was clear: it hadn't, in fact, been necessary to remove the second testicle.

I felt that sinking sensation somewhere deep inside me again but maintained my sang-froid. Perhaps most guys would have made a fuss at this point, but it seemed to me that getting all emotional wouldn't really help anybody. Anyway, I'd resolved to get through this in as dignified a manner as possible, and I darned well was going to see it through. I numbly, dumbly listened as the surgeon told me that this sort of situation was unavoidable, that it was just one of those unfortunate things that happened sometimes.

A registrar from the Oncology team took a very different view. At the first out-patient appointment following my second orchidectomy, her exact words to me were – "this shouldn't have happened". It seemed a bit late to do anything about it now though. In the days and weeks afterwards, my friends suggested that I had solid grounds to make a complaint. I felt uncomfortable that they were angry on my behalf when I just wanted the whole thing to be over and put it all behind me. I didn't want to deal with difficult emotions so I just put a lid on them instead and screwed it down as tightly as I could. The hidden black hole underwent a real growth spurt as a result.

Stiff upper lip, chin up, crack on. I was going to act like a man, even though I wasn't one anymore. I didn't complain, but I didn't ever get on with my life either, as it turned out. Everyone seemed impressed with how well I dealt with the illness and operations, but I wasn't dealing with any of it at all. An ex-girlfriend suggested that I was in denial – I denied this quite firmly. She was right of course; too bad it took me over twenty years to realise it.

Whilst I had been going through the tests and operations, I hadn't really considered how things would be afterwards. I just assumed that I was going to be impotent but discovered that this was not necessarily the case.

In April I was put on male hormone replacement therapy – testosterone injections. After starting these, I experienced "hot flushes", then one morning woke up to a pleasant surprise – an erection, my first in a while.

I would later discover that orgasms feel a bit different without balls. I was literally "firing blanks" now, but at least the "gun" was in some sort of operating order again. Most of the ejaculate fluid that a man shoots when he orgasms is produced by the prostate gland, the testicles only contribute sperm to the mix. Life went on, it usually does. Now I was back at work and everything was going to return to normal once more. Wasn't it?

Every month for a year, and for several years after that with less frequency, I had check-ups to make sure there was no secondary spread of malignancy. It seemed unlikely to me that this would happen, as the primary site of malignancy had been removed. From the first day, I never felt I was in any danger of dying. I never experienced any "battle" with cancer. The conflict that I would fight was to be a cold war within myself over the next two decades.

It didn't take long before I was struck by the first poison darts of mockery, each one leaving no external mark but spreading its venom inside me, hidden from view.

Someone at work thought it was funny to address me in a high-pitched voice. I wondered if I should smash his face in, but I didn't. I didn't do anything. A former manager visited my department at the hospital; his wife was attending for an appointment. I asked him if he was enjoying his retirement, he smirked and asked me if I was enjoying mine. At first, I didn't know what he meant, but his nasty smile made it clear to me. At a social event a drunken lady, who worked at the hospital, referred to a nearby pool table and said I couldn't play because I didn't have any balls. Cricket and football provide many opportunities for jokes about balls, and the lack of them. Maybe I'm too sensitive; perhaps I should just toughen up a bit. Sticks and stones…but words can hurt too. Each jibe caused a scar that never heals.

You get a year to complain about something in the NHS. Over a year after my operations, a friend told me that she'd read an item in the local paper that might interest me and sent a cutting to me through the post. It reported on a case that was being heard at Crown Court: a man had one of his testicles removed following a misdiagnosis at the same hospital as me. An ultrasound scan had indicated malignancy, but after the testicle was removed it was found that no cancer had been present. The court heard evidence that ultrasound scans were sometimes known to give "false positive" results in such cases. The consultant radiologist who gave evidence on behalf of the hospital stated that such cases were extremely rare and that they'd had no similar ones before or since. That seemed to be possibly rather like a misleading statement to me. It was as if the hospital was saying that what had happened to me hadn't really happened at all. The other man's misdiagnosis had occurred only a short time apart from mine – two such "highly atypical" probabilities occurring so closely together in isolation seemed to be stretching credibility a little too far perhaps. I pushed down on the sinking sensation that rose up inside me again, inadvertently providing more nourishment for the black hole to feast upon.

Ever since that late-night trip to the toilet before that particular Christmas, I had pretended that everything was fine. Everything wasn't fine though, something was very wrong, but I didn't know what. Perhaps I do now. I very much wish that I was able to go back and have a good long conversation with my younger self – I would have some hard-learnt wisdom to share with that naive, well-intentioned softie. I would impress upon him the importance of feelings, of being emotionally literate, and having the courage to admit weakness and vulnerability. I would tell him that it was vital that he love himself, tell him not to be afraid, and that he must not let fear dictate his actions (or lack of actions). Maybe that's all that he needed someone to tell him. But no-one ever did, and it's too late now.

A few years ago, I requested a copy of my hospital notes, paying the required fee. When I read through them, I discovered that the Consultant Oncologist had written to the Consultant Surgeon twice to suggest that a biopsy should be carried out on my left testicle before it was removed. I wish I'd known that then…

I attempted to complain to the hospital about my misdiagnosis twenty years ago, but was brushed off by them. I had hoped that they might provide me with some counselling perhaps, but the Chief Executive wrote to me and suggested that I should go and see my GP if I was experiencing any issues relating to the matter.

You could say that the sperm I banked all those years ago didn't accrue any interest and the account has now been closed. When I reached 55 years of age it was destroyed in accordance with the relevant legislation. My genes will never be passed on any further – good news for humanity.

I must be one of the few people to have lost three balls; two natural, and one artificial. As Oscar Wilde *might* have said – to lose one testicle may be regarded as a misfortune; to lose both looks like carelessness. I wonder what he would have said about a hat-trick – doubtless something very witty.

The black hole continued growing inside me. One day it overflowed, and I became lost in darkness.

Hello

I knew someone would come along, and I'm glad that it turned out to be you. I think that perhaps everything will be okay now.

People like me don't write books, but I have tried my best all the same. My "literary" background is in music fanzines – made with glue and scissors in the true "cut'n'paste" tradition. My little 'zine soon became too big and mutated into this sprawling album of weirdness. You may wonder why anyone would attempt a task that they are so ill-equipped to fulfil. The only answer I can give is – because I had to.

For many, many years there was a hidden darkness concealed deep within me. I tried to ignore it, but this only allowed the black hole to grow further, until it overwhelmed me, and I *became* the black hole. And then, suddenly, the emotions that I had locked away securely within myself for several years were released in a massive psychological jailbreak. All the grief and pain that I had imprisoned now overwhelmed me. By putting myself in a deep-freeze, I had postponed the reckoning but now it was here, and it was going to hurt – a lot. The brittle creation of the self I sought to be had broken under pressure, the pieces were now scattered widely. I picked some of them up, but they made no sense; I couldn't tell how they fitted together – or even if they did fit together in any way.

There is an old Swahili proverb – to get lost is to find the way. I sought to discover something that was concealed in plain sight. Was there a little lost voice coming from my own personal Pandora's Box that I could hear? It was faint, but there was definitely something. I wanted to express myself but didn't know what to say. I wanted to tell a story but didn't know what it was. For the first time in my life I began to think about who I was, and what I could be, not what I was supposed to be. I had been closed off and shut down for many years. Now I had been blown wide open and there was nowhere to hide.

I began writing, attempting to record the thoughts and feelings that began to fizz through me. I drained the void onto reams of paper via the ink from many pens. Distracted scribbles were transferred to a keyboard, and then gradually became the banal and broken kaleidoscope that you are about to discover.

I have found this to be a difficult process. Apart from the discomfort caused by exploring distressing places within yourself, there is the elusiveness of the truth itself. After you have meticulously stripped away a layer of self-deception, pain may suggest that you have touched the truth. Later you realise that there is, in fact, another transparent layer of unconscious deceit that you must, with unflinching patience, peel off. Often there are many layers that must be removed before there are none left, and you have finally reached what you seek. In the past I often mistook vicious self-criticism for truthfulness, but self-hatred is only another type of deception that will stop you finding wisdom and self-knowledge. So, I will tell my story as well as I can, avoiding any temptation to portray myself in a flattering light.

I did think about paying an English Literature student to re-write all this nonsense and see if they could make it readable. Then I realised that it wouldn't be mine anymore if this happened, it might even become something legitimate – a proper writer's idea of what I'm trying to say. I felt it had to be ugly and poorly realised for it to be true, it had to have little or no value for it to be worth anything.

I began picking up the pieces, discarding those that did not fit with the new inchoate me that was slowly coalescing into existence. I wanted to invent a new and improved Laurence but remained unsure how to fit the pieces together. So, I have laid the fragments out carefully, hoping that someday someone might see hidden messages concealed in my unpromising mosaic. Stories that might tell me about myself, and perhaps reveal something to you about yourself too. I worry that perhaps there are no secrets waiting to be revealed though; maybe there is truly nothing there at all. Yet even nothing is something sometimes.

Somehow, I have ended up here.

Randomness has played a significant role in the order of items; this scrapbook is an ever-changing collection, and this edition can be considered a "snap-shot" of material that is in continuous flux. It seems to me that this kind of layout is the most sensible way to express the fragmentary nature of the hidden world where these postcards have been sent from.

You can read this jumble of words any way that suits you. Start at the beginning and work your way through to the end, or dip in and out randomly – you decide. You might also perhaps wish to leave now, having seen quite enough already. That's fine too; you will depart with no hard feelings and my best wishes. For what is coming isn't going to be to everyone's liking, I'm afraid. I tried to steer the material in certain directions, but it was too strong for me. In the end, the material chose its own path and I was merely a helpless passenger trapped on a runaway vehicle.

I would be pleased if you chose to stay a while. I really need someone to be on my side and would be pleased if you were. Anyway, thank you for being here.

unsung love song

A Wretched Gift

I wish that I could offer you something more beautiful
and full of hope; but all I can give is my bitterness and
regrets, my twisted heart and my poisoned soul. These
may still be of greater value than they might at first seem,
for I hope that you will gain light from my darkness. I
ask that you learn from me and do not be as I was.

If my ugliness can make you more aware of your
beauty, my foolishness teach you wisdom, my weakness
show you your strength – then my poor offering may
prove much more valuable than the sum of its sorry parts.

Jigsaw

You pick up a piece and vaguely consider whether it
might fit somewhere. You have a box that's full of many
assorted pieces but there is no picture to guide you.
Anyway, it's obvious that all the pieces can't fit together
as they're plainly from many different puzzles – at least
that's how it seems. You keep finding pieces in the
oddest and most unexpected places too, and sometimes
a single piece appears to be a complete story by itself.
Somehow, an obscure sense can be made when you

randomly gather a few pieces and place them together without thinking about it too much. It seems more beautiful that way, even if it you don't understand why.

The Shame

My kind has disgusted normal people for many centuries. The earliest records of our existence come from the ancient Sumerian city of Lagash, in what is now known as Iraq, and these date from the twenty-first century BCE. Perhaps we were around before then too, inviting contempt and disdain. We live in the shadows, beyond the fringes of acceptability, furtively seeking small moments of happiness. Still we dream of walking in the light with our heads held high, and who knows…perhaps one fine day?

Spadone

It's pronounced "spay-dun" and is the name that's sometimes given to eunuchs who have had their testicles removed but whose penis remains intact. This was the method of castration practiced in the Persian empires – the penis was left in place to avoid urinary problems. The term has been used in the past to describe sexually abstinent men as well as eunuchs.

In Imperial China eunuchs had their penises removed as well as their testicles, as was also the case with African eunuchs who served in the Ottoman Empire. Castrato singers and European Byzantine eunuchs normally had their penises left in place.

A Few Different Post-Castration Names

Cat: gib
Cattle: 1. bullock (when testicles are removed
      whilst immature – also "steer" in US)
    2. ox (when testicles are removed in
      adulthood)
Chicken: capon
Goat and sheep: wether
Horse: gelding
Human: eunuch
Pig: 1. barrow (when testicles are removed whilst
    immature)
    2. stag (when testicles are removed in
      adulthood)

Oddly, perhaps, there is no specific term for dogs that have been neutered.

Music as Life Support

There are times in life when music may become a necessity. When I was lost in the darkness, I found that music could reach deep inside and make me feel alive instead of being numb. I went to almost a hundred and twenty gigs one year, plus a couple of festivals. Going to live music performances became a compulsion, and a therapy. Music was a healing experience when I was in a critical emotional state. I would close my eyes and let the sounds overwhelm me; they would soak through the cracks in my physical shell and nourish my ailing spirit. I became lost within the music, and then sometimes I'd *become* the music for just a little while. I was picked up and carried away on coloured waves, floated in the air above, then was placed gently back upon earth once more, a little better for the trip.

I was brought up a Catholic and couldn't avoid making spiritual and religious comparisons to the conduct of a gig. The stage was like an altar, the performers the celebrants of the mass, and the audience the congregation.

I attended many gigs, shows and concerts and noted them down with a cricket-scorer's thoroughness. Then, one March, without realising it at the time, I stopped suddenly. I was healed, or at least a stage of recovery had been completed. Where before I'd been hollow and flimsy, after a slow process of growth I had become stronger and acquired an internal substance. I had eventually developed into a new version of me somehow. I still go to gigs but with far less frequency than I used to.

Babel-onia

Manchester is a big dump really; a dirty, litter-strewn blot upon the Earth – but I have an affection for it all the same. It has been suggested that no city in the United Kingdom had its head further up its own backside, whilst some of its natives claim it to be a superior place above all others. Each year the universities draw in a new wave of youthful talent and creative energy which greatly enriches the city. People come from many faraway lands to work and live here, helping the city to grow further. Research suggests that up to two hundred languages might be spoken here.

Coffee Shops

I visit many coffee shops, even though I no longer drink coffee. I can't sleep if I have just one cup earlier in the day. I still greatly enjoy tea, however, and appreciate a pot of a good loose-leaf blend very much – especially when accompanied by a delicious slice of cake. Whilst it is important that such places sell quality beverages and food, there are other elements that make a coffee shop worth visiting. A good coffee shop sells more than coffee, tea and cakes – it provides an experience. You must feel that you have come home when you enter, the atmosphere within must be relaxing yet also offer gentle sensory and emotional stimulation. There must be a feeling of acceptance – a good place brings warmth to the heart, is somewhere that you might find stillness whilst surrounded by movement.

Coffee shops are resting places for those exploring the urban expanse, staging posts for travellers making journeys or pilgrimages. They are refuges to pause for a short time, collect thoughts and restore equilibrium. They provide a place to meet, to hide or disappear briefly, to re-gather composure and strength, to consider important matters in a calm manner.

I mapped the city on lost wanderings and committed my surveys to paper in coffee shops. Each is a relay station where trivial but potentially precious observations can be recorded on paper before they are forgotten by a fading brain.

Cai Lun

Cai Lun was a eunuch and an official of the Han court. The imperial bureaucracy generated a great deal of "paperwork" before there was such a thing as paper, when documents were written on bamboo or silk. Cai Lun is credited with inventing paper and the paper-making process about 1,900 years ago. One story suggests that he drew inspiration from watching paper-wasps build their nest. His innovation transformed Chinese culture and education, eventually spreading across the world. He was awarded honours and wealth for his invention but after a change of Emperor, committed suicide rather than be imprisoned.

12 and 3 makes Infinity

The three chord, twelve bar form may be amongst the human race's greatest artistic achievements. So simple that anyone can play it, yet providing infinite space for expression. Within this simple construction, the great are equal with the lowest. It's a place where it's not what you do that's important, it's the *way* you do it.

Superhero Power

If you could have one superhero power, what would you choose? I rather like the idea of being able to understand and communicate in any language. Such a gift might seem prosaic compared to some that you could think of, but it's the one that appeals to me most. Imagine being able to talk with anyone. I struggle with one language, as you may have noticed. I think it's amazing that some people can understand several languages and switch between them without hesitation.

The Neutered Gaze

I look at women more than I ever did when I was a complete man. Usually I observe them in an abstract, disconnected way; it may register with me that a particular lady is very attractive, but I won't *feel* any desire for her. It's like turning on a switch, but the relevant appliance doesn't work; the light doesn't come on, the power doesn't start, there is no operational mechanism. Sometimes I desperately press the switch and despair at what has been lost to me forever.

I also look at a woman sometimes and am overcome by a deep sadness. She reminds me of my pointlessness, my ugliness, my lack of worth. I cannot feel desire as normal men do; consequently, my appreciation of women is more subtle and intense for its impossible and inexpressible nature. I may not have any balls, nor a fully functioning dick, but other aspects of my being work well enough. I am far more sensitive to subtle evocations of femininity than I ever was when I was a man.

The Lo-Fi Sound of Illegible Scribbles

I have the writer's equivalent of three chords and an out-of-tune guitar. I've something to say, if not a vocabulary to express it. I will make a glorious racket of freak-show weirdness and scribble a series of short postcards from a strange place. I'll record on a wobbly old analogue 4-track and make a handful of demo cassettes that I'll give away to random people who aren't really interested at all. Nobody will ever listen to them, and it will all have been for nothing. All the same, I must do it.

Kevin Briggs

Kevin is a retired highway patrolman who served in California. The area he patrolled included the Golden Gate Bridge, which crosses San Francisco Bay, and is one of the most famous suicide spots in the world. As soon as he started working in the area, he found himself talking to people who had climbed over the safety rail and were considering ending their lives. Even though he had received no training he would try to talk them out of jumping. He usually asked them how they were doing and what their plans were for tomorrow, then he'd listen. It's estimated that he dissuaded a couple of hundred people from taking their own lives. He now gives talks on suicide prevention.

Taking Pictures

I take pictures on my walks around the city; not proper photographs, but "point and press" snaps. I have an auto-focus camera and it's pretty much idiot-proof, but I still manage to take the most awful pictures – a five year-old could take better ones. I try to capture flux, to document change, such as buildings being constructed or demolished and neighbourhoods undergoing transformations. Often, I'll take a series of pictures that show a location altering subtly over time. I also like to catch fleeting, forgotten moments and conjunctions that probably no-one was ever aware of. Most of my pictures are very boring. There are two other subjects that I try and catch. I like to take pictures of other people taking pictures of the city, and I like to capture couples walking along the street holding hands. These both involve some surreptitious snapping as people have then become the subject instead of being an incidental feature, as is the case when you take a picture of a street, building or a landscape.

Unplayed Memories

I owned the complete Postcard Records catalogue but hadn't played any of the releases for several years. I took them to a Northern Quarter record shop and sold them. I could have made more by selling them myself through appropriate websites, but this would have taken an amount of time and effort that I didn't want to waste upon such a task. The records themselves meant nothing to me anymore, although I still have a sense of nostalgia for the times when these bands were around – when I was young, and life was full of wonderful possibilities. You actually believed, then, that a new seven-inch single could change everything – the sweet foolishness of youth. Now I realise that bands I once admired were pretentious posers, little more than disposable commodities in a cynical business, exploiting impressionable consumers like me.

Deterrence

I remember one evening in the mid to late 1970s, I watched an interview on television. The format was simple; the camera pointed at the subject, who spoke to an interviewer that was off-screen, the background was darkness – at least that's how I recall it forty years later. I can't remember the name of the programme, the man talking was from Glasgow, I think. He spoke about his heroin addiction; he explained about the feeling of the rush when the drug had been injected. He also explained the degradations and humiliations that his addiction had led him into. He wept when he described being at his daughter's funeral and being so wasted that he had little idea where he was. It was a powerful piece of television that had a great effect upon me. The man said that if even one person was dissuaded from using drugs after listening to him speak then his life would not have been in vain. At the end of the film a message stated that the man had died shortly after recording had been completed.

The Parable of the Talents

You've heard this before? The master leaves for a while, entrusting some of his wealth to three servants. Two trade at a market and earn further wealth, whilst the third buries his share so that it will be safe. The master returns and is angry at the third servant who allowed fear to dictate his actions; he did not make use of what he had been given.

I used to wonder how it would have been received if one of the servants had taken the wealth entrusted to him, traded unsuccessfully and lost it all. What would the master have said to that? Eventually I realised that this would have been impossible. The teller of the parable was attempting to explain that if each individual uses whatever abilities they are given in a positive manner, then an increase in value is inevitable. Those who cravenly hide their potential and do not develop the abilities that they have been given will suffer greatly. Fear is the enemy that kills you from the inside – negativity is poison.

One aspect of the parable that is rarely considered is that the master entrusts the servants with varying amounts "each according to his ability". The servant who failed the master's test was the least gifted; perhaps there is a suggestion that those with lower worth are less likely to succeed in life.

Pornography

I had never seen a porn movie until I was thirty-six. I was experiencing a high sex drive, with constant erections at the time – something I can only dream of now. At first, when I viewed these sorts of movies, I felt conflicting responses. I was bemused, appalled and aroused by what I saw. I watched, puzzled, asking myself – "why are they doing that?" Porn creates its own language and filters out many of the things that make sex wonderful, then turbo-charges a narrow part of the carnal spectrum relentlessly. Once you've tuned into the wavelength of this distorted signal it can become very compelling. For me, porn and reality were clearly distinct areas, separated by a wide boundary. I had no wish to act out in real life what I watched; it was fantasy. It wasn't my fantasy though. It was a degraded synthetic product, and I began consuming it in the absence of any other alternative. My natural, personal fantasies about women were absurdly tame and I felt very guilty about being aroused by some of the staples of porn. Mainstream hardcore usually shows women being used roughly and suggests that this is the baseline for normal intercourse. As I had no other means of sexual expression, I began to use porn with increasing regularity. If I felt attracted to a woman in the real world, it caused me pain; a toxic backdraft of shame, inadequacy and self-hatred overwhelmed me. Porn numbed difficult feelings, anaesthetised awkward emotions. It was the arousal itself that was compelling, not the sweet release. The neural pathways inside my head lit up with a glowing, artificial incandescence, and my brain melted into a thick, sweet syrup. My body was pumped and hot, my heart pounded. I forgot everything else, my consciousness reduced to a small area of delicious heat throbbing under an intense and ecstatic light. I kept shaking the bottle to increase the fizziness; opening it brought an overwhelming release that was only temporary. It was the hyped-up effervescence that I craved, I felt very alive in this aroused state – a compelling illusion when parts of you are dead, but the energy goes nowhere, brings no benefit, can only feed off itself. It was an exquisite torture that I greedily embraced. Like Sisyphus pushing the boulder up the slope, I became enslaved by the pointlessness itself. When the stone rolled back to the bottom, I was glad because now I could begin all over again and be consumed once more by the enchanting illusion of pleasure. I used pornography to overcome low self-esteem and psychological suffering but ended up becoming lost in a cycle of regret, shame, and self-loathing that only made things worse.

The formulaic nature of the material is repetitive; the regular viewer desires a reliably predictable experience, yet at the same time wants it to feel new. There are various aspects of fantasy – some things you would like to act out in real life, but others you only wish to experience inside your head. Fantasising about something does not indicate a wish for it to become real. Some suggest that romantic fantasies, as portrayed in films and books, are a kind of emotional pornography. People enjoy all sorts of film fantasies that aren't erotic in nature – action, science-fiction, horror, and many other genres. Enjoying these doesn't mean that the viewer wishes to actually be placed in the situations portrayed within them. Fantasy can skew perceptions, distorting reality. Porn is a lie that pretends to be fun. It isn't.

Castrato Singers

In 1588 the Pope banned women from singing in public. This led to the practice of young boys being castrated before their voices broke so that they could sing soprano vocal parts previously performed by women. Poor families sometimes castrated their sons in the hope that they would go on to lucrative careers and be able to support them; this was not always the case, unfortunately. Castration before puberty prevents the larynx from developing normally and the voice from "breaking", producing a unique quality. It also causes bone epiphyses to remain softer and often castrati had long limbs. In addition, this also sometimes produced more supple ribcages and castrati often had powerful lung capacities. As a result of this, and small child-like vocal cords, the resultant singing voice could be extremely flexible and have a great range. With training, a beautiful instrument might be developed but many boys didn't turn out to be talented singers and lived a miserable existence in adulthood. Sometimes women pretended to be castrati so that they could have the opportunity to sing that the church had attempted to deny them.

A few castrati achieved enormous success and consequently gained much female attention, leading to unusual assignations and relationships. They were treated like rock stars and celebrities are today. Probably the most famous and admired was Farinelli, who is also counted as one of the greatest opera singers ever. Nowadays, Moreschi is probably the better known, even though he was considered an undistinguished singer, as he was the only castrati to make solo recordings. These were made in 1902 when castrati were becoming rarer, the Italian government having banned castration in 1870.

Down at the Bottom of the Food Chain

I survive upon the smallest morsels. I do not feast upon the crumbs that fall from the tables of the blessed and the beautiful but scavenge upon those that have been crushed underfoot into the dirt. I am deformed by loneliness, twisted by shame, tormented by sweet dreams of what might have been and bitter regrets for what came to be. If an attractive woman is pleasant to me, even just briefly, I will treasure it in my heart long afterwards.

Psychological Antibiotics

Untreated infections fester and spread, causing great damage. I obstinately denied myself basic care for years, causing increased suffering. Too proud, too ignorant, I put my faith in making problems disappear by pretending they didn't exist. Eventually, I conceded that I had been my own worst enemy and began treatment. The prescription was contained in books and people, music and city streets, and also within my heart. At first the effects were minimal, but you must complete the entire course for it to be effective, you cannot skip part of the whole. Now I am healing, the fever that once seemed normal has receded, my strength increases slowly.

Performance

When I was young, I believed that records were better than live music. A recording was the perfect realisation of the artist's vision which could be appreciated fully at the listener's convenience. Often, I went to gigs and was disappointed that bands seemed to produce poor versions of their recordings on stage. The audience also became a distraction from listening properly too.

Nowadays, I feel it is the other way around. Live performance is to be in the moment, to share a common experience. It is "now", and then it is gone forever. Music is better with "mistakes" and irregularities – perfection is bland.

The Cowardly Hero

When I saw *The Magnificent Seven* as a youngster, I was not particularly impressed by Lee. He was the gunman who had lost his nerve and was fighting a battle within himself, whilst most of his colleagues were displaying the traditional ideals of masculine courage. Now, I think he's the most interesting character in the film, and perhaps, in some ways, the bravest one, because he confronted the fear that was destroying him. Robert Vaughn's portrayal of the flawed man, trying to conceal his weakness behind a firm-jawed mask which had slipped a little was perfect. Many will feel distaste and contempt for a character whose inner conflict was tearing him apart, but now that I understand his situation better, I'm on his side.

Red Thread

An eastern Asian myth which suggests that the gods fasten an invisible red thread around a limb of those destined to meet and love each other later in life. It may stretch and tangle but can never break. Perhaps not everyone has one though.

Lunchtime Recital

During late autumn, winter, and early spring, the RNCM (Royal Northern College of Music) puts on free lunch-time concerts where students perform a wide range of works. On Mondays it's usually a recital by a solo performer or small ensembles, and on Thursdays something orchestral. I always enjoy attending these events. One season a bit of a crèche developed, where up to five mothers brought along babies or very young children. It wasn't much of a distraction if one of the babies began crying, it was almost part of the performance.

Funny

Women like guys who have a sense of humour, but I'm not much of comedian; when I try to tell a joke it always falls flat. The only time I get a laugh is when I'm attempting to impress people with my intelligence or making a misguided effort to appear cool – then I'm *really* hilarious.

Nonentity

Nowadays you often hear about LGBTI – Lesbian, Gay, Bisexual, Transsexual/Transgender, Intersex. In the most sexualised culture in human history we are presented with more identities and less distinct boundaries between them than ever before. Even this wider acceptance and understanding doesn't cover the full range of possibilities, though. Transsex suggests a dynamic of going somewhere, it has a destination. Intersex suggests a place, a newly discovered land that is home to those who belong there, perhaps a slender isthmus between two continents. A eunuch is just nothing; a pointlessness stripped of any worth and value. Whilst I may desperately wish to think in conventional terms about what I am and would like to be, this can never correspond with the physical reality. The eunuch identity carries no status; they are gender nonentities, invisible on the sexual spectrum, living in an eternal state of disgrace. Facebook apparently now has fifty-six options for members' gender, but some people don't fit any of them. It seems that literally I may be a big fat nothing.

Walking

It's what the human body was designed to do, the reason for our upright gait. Sometimes when I'm down or agitated I go for a long walk and feel much better afterwards. I read about a lady whose son was in a coma in Intensive Care; she spent as much time as she could with him, but each day went for a long walk in the city surrounding the hospital – she said it kept her sane. I began walking after reading her story.

Sometimes I stroll slowly, sometimes I stride a little quicker; only robots walk at the same pace all the time. Sometimes my steps are confident and certain, at other times indecisive and unsure. Sometimes I watch everything very closely, noting tiny details, at other times my unfocused gaze causes the city to become a blur that washes over me. Sometimes I have a clear destination in mind, sometimes I have no idea where I'm going but still arrive somewhere. I may seek out little backstreets and alleys that are new to me, or travel through familiar routes that change every day in sometimes barely perceptible ways. After a while, my body settles into a comfortably repetitive movement and my jammed-up mind begins to turn over smoothly, impossible puzzles soon begin to make sense somehow.

Hopeless

When I saw a counsellor, he advised me to avoid online dating and speed dating, in fact anything with a "date" aspect, as I would only be setting myself up to fail. He said I was a five-out-of-ten, and women are looking for eight-out-of-tens. That might sound a bit brutal, but I was grateful for his honesty. He suggested that it would be better to acquire a social circle which included potentially suitable women. I could make friends with ladies, and this might perhaps lead to more if there was a mutual attraction. For a reclusive misfit like me, this would be very difficult though as I don't really have a social circle. Let's face it, finding women who might be interested in me would be a needle-in-a-haystack scenario anyway. I was crushed when he suggested that I call Silverline, a 'phone service for lonely old people. I knew then that there was no hope left for me.

Saint Ignatius of Constantinople

He was son of the Emperor, but when his father was deposed, he was forcibly castrated, which meant that he was ineligible to ever become Emperor himself – a eunuch could not claim this position. He was incarcerated in a monastery, took to the religious life and was made an abbot. Later he was appointed Patriarch of Constantinople. In this role he was embroiled in many political and religious issues of the day, particularly relating to iconoclasm and jurisdiction over the newly-converted Bulgaria, as well as the debauched behaviour prevalent in the imperial court at that time. This brought him into conflict with both the Emperor and the Pope, and he was deposed but reappointed some years later. Recognised as a saint by the Roman Catholic Church, his feast day is the 23rd of October. Other eunuch saints of Byzantium were Saint Germanus and Saint Methodius.

Fully Equipped

I always carry a few items in my pockets or in my rucksack when I wander around the city; I find they come in useful sometimes. These include:

A few pens, good ones (I personally dislike using pencils)

A small pocket notebook, ring-bound with easy-to-tear-off pages

A larger A4 writing pad in my rucksack

An A to Z of Manchester

A camera, nowadays most younger people use their 'phone instead

Earplugs, for noisy environments, also last-minute surprise gigs

Paper tissues in my rucksack – handy things to have

Usually I have toothpaste and a toothbrush in my rucksack, sometimes I have a little toiletries bag as well

A lighter (even though I don't smoke myself)

Clean handkerchiefs

Reading glasses (more than one pair – I've lost a few before)

Whichever book I'm currently plodding my way through

A hopeful heart, an open mind, and a sharp eye (on a good day)

Money to buy tea and cake, pay for car parking or transport, and to give to those that may need a little bit of help

Northern Quarter Dream

There are a few record shops in the NQ, but no real bookshops. If I won the lottery, I'd open up a place that covered several floors and was a proper independent bookstore, which would be staffed by book lovers. I'd also like to have a really good coffee and tea shop on the premises, and a small performance space where music gigs and book events could take place. I like fantasising about this imaginary enterprise – it would operate at a loss, but it would be the most special and wonderful place to visit, and everyone who came in the door would leave enriched by the experience.

Summer of Love

Some music historians may suggest that 1977 was the year that punk overthrew the oppressors of big business, in a grass-roots revolution that changed everything for-ever. It wasn't really like that, but everyone has myths that they hold dear. 'Hotel California' by The Eagles was a massive hit that year, but it was another big seller that heralded a new dawn more powerfully than any contrived, back-to-basics bandwagon. The sound of that summer was Donna Summer's 'I Feel Love' – the work of producer Giorgio Moroder and Pete Bellote. Gleamingly sensuous electronica, relentless programmed rhythms draped with layers of hazy desire. It was the sound of the future.

Note to Self

What a shit you are – feeling sorry for yourself whilst other people have *real* problems in life, and deal with them with a humility and dignity that's far beyond you. Get your head out of your arse, you selfish, self-absorbed loser.

Sleeping Together

I have spent every night of this century alone and fully accept that I am unlikely to be an attractive prospect for any lady to share a bed with. I remember before I was castrated, when I had girlfriends. I enjoyed cuddling them before they went to sleep and cuddling them again in the morning. There is something wonderfully intimate about sleeping together — just sleeping beside each other. Sometimes I would wake up during the night and listen to her breathing whilst she slept, or I would wake first in the morning and look at her as she lay beside me. At such times I always felt that I was lucky, but even then, I didn't know how fortunate I was.

A Faded Monochrome Rainbow

A great part of the erotic spectrum has, for me, been obliterated by castration, but a seedling under paving stones will try to find a crack through which it might reach towards the light. It will be stunted and distorted when it emerges from the concrete, but whilst it lives it will hope. I was never much given to coarse carnality in any case; I was too much of a nice-boy square for that, was too repressed to allow myself to be consumed by lust whilst I was still physically capable of expressing it. Now it hurts if I feel attracted to a woman, which I still occasionally do, as strong feelings of worthlessness and inadequacy soon follow and overwhelm me. I still very much cherish women though, even more so in some ways. Perhaps small fragments of the spectrum still remain and have become enhanced in an attempt to compensate for that which has been lost. I deeply appreciate the way some women dress, their demeanour, subtle expressions of individuality. Slight, unconscious gestures have a powerful effect. Small unrealised mannerisms bring much delight. I have always valued such things, but now I'm even more intensely aware of these than before.

Femininity is only an invention conjured by our minds, a creation of the collective consciousness. If that's the case, then it's one of the human race's best ideas, I think.

Eunuchs in the Imperial Court of China

For centuries in Imperial China, castration was used as a punishment, but could also be a passport to employment in the imperial palace. Men who did not belong to the imperial family were rarely permitted within the boundaries of the Forbidden City, but eunuchs were; they served in a wide range of roles within this secretive place. Eunuchs were regarded as lacking aggression and ambition, as well as having no sexual potency. This made them perfect attendants and administrators and ensured that there was no possible impropriety with the imperial concubines. They were also viewed by many as being venal and calculating and were greatly despised. Living within this private world allowed privileged access to the Emperor and presented the opportunity to influence decisions, therefore acquiring a degree of power as a consequence. Chinese eunuchs had their

penises cut off as well as their testicles, without anaesthetic and with negligible consideration for hygiene.
They were prone to chronic and painful urinary infections, and many became incontinent as they grew older
and wore a nappy beneath their outer clothing, causing
them to smell and be the subject of even further disdain – "smell like a eunuch" was a common insult. The
imperial eunuchs had to submit to an annual inspec-
tion to confirm their lack of genitalia. Often eunuchs
attempted to run away from court due to the mistreat-
ment they received, and were punished harshly when
caught, whilst others realised that they would never meet
with anything but contempt outside the palace – there
were many suicides. Most eunuchs were illiterate, but
some were very well educated. During various dynas-
ties the eunuch population numbered many thousands,
but by the early twentieth century their numbers had
dwindled to just several hundred in the palace. Many
eunuchs had "dining partners" – a term used for relationships within the court between two women, or a
eunuch and a woman. Unofficial marriages took place
between eunuchs and palace women, some adopted
children, and others associated with prostitutes and conducted secret relationships with them. Attractive young
eunuchs sometimes became subject to the sexual atten-
tions of male members of the royal family.

Anatoly Koryagin

He was a doctor who protested about the use of psychiatric hospitals to imprison dissidents. He was himself sentenced to hard labour, and told the court at his trial that he would never accept that trying to think independently was a mental illness, and a crime punishable by detention. He went on hunger strike and was force-fed; he was administered antipsychotic drugs and beaten, but he did not break.

There have been many ordinary people who have stood up to overwhelmingly oppressive regimes whose heroism is unknown and forgotten. There are some who are prepared to speak up and stand against what is evil and wrong. We are lucky that there are such people in the world, because we desperately need them.

'Phone a Friend

I had no-one to talk to. Isolation was crushing me, so I called a 'phone sex service. I spoke to some ladies regularly and, in a strange way, became attached to them. Some of them were very smart and clever women, who had done a lot of interesting things in the past and had some unusual perspectives. I still think about them occasionally and hope that they are happy. At the darkest times in my life, the only people I had to confide in were these ladies. Some worked in the service for only a few months, whilst others did so for years. I found myself listening to stories from their lives too, it took me out of myself – their tales were much more interesting than mine. The longer the conversation, the more money they made. I'm sure that they probably wouldn't have wasted any time talking to me had they not been paid to do so, but I was still shown kindness by these ladies and I'm grateful to them for this.

Turning Back from the Edge

I took the stairs to the top level; there were hardly any cars. I walked through the wide concrete space to the back, where it might be done. I had haunted this place many times before in dark torments of the mind, and now, for the first time, I was actually here. I leant over the barrier and looked at the ground below. It was high enough. Headfirst, to be certain. Many times, I had imagined how it would be – the ending. Now that I could feel the rail on my hand and the breeze upon my face, it wasn't real.

A door banged behind me, it echoed loudly. I turned around, a man with a black plastic sack, collecting litter. He looked at me, wondering what I was doing. Yes, what was I doing? I looked back out over the city, when I turned around again, he'd gone. I decided, turned towards the stairs. I knew that I wasn't going to do it.

Unsociable

I wouldn't say that I suffer from social anxiety, but I'm certainly not very comfortable when meeting people and interacting with them. Perhaps I underwent a charisma bypass procedure once; I lack confidence, am dull and uninteresting. I feel awkward and out of place in social situations, I make banal and tedious conversation, my body language is stiff and ungainly. Perhaps for a few minutes I can hold up my end of a discussion with someone, but soon feel a dread rise inside me, and often guillotine the exchange by saying I have to go somewhere. At other times, I attempt to compensate by chattering idiotically, and later cringe with embarrassment when I realise how stupid I must have appeared. I enjoy being amongst people but can feel detached from them, that I do not belong with them, even though I would very much like to. I have a solitary aspect to my nature but also feel very isolated and lonely too sometimes.

Jia Xian

A Chinese eunuch and mathematician of the eleventh century century who invented Pascal's Triangle – six hundred years before Pascal himself did so. This is used to calculate square and cubic roots. He wrote a book explaining his theories, but no copies survive.

Vicarious Pleasure

Sometimes I sit and watch people passing by in town. I particularly enjoy observing couples walking along with their arms linked or holding hands. I like to see their smiling faces, hear their enraptured voices, and experience a second-hand happiness by witnessing theirs. I am pleased to know that love is actually out there, and occasionally when I see a pair consumed with a particularly appealing blend of mutual delight and amazement, I feel a small moment of diluted joy within me.

Dating

I've dated four ladies in the last five years, without getting as far as a third date with any of them. Dating when you're old can be quite a disheartening experience. It seems to be really difficult to meet nice women around my age. They must be out there somewhere though, mustn't they?

Abelard

A distinguished academic in twelfth century France, he fell in love with Heloise – it was a forbidden romance. Her uncle arranged for a gang to break into

Abelard's chamber whilst he slept and castrate him; Heloise had already given birth to a child and took refuge in a convent. Abelard later became a monk and lived in a monastery. There are disputes about where the ill-starred couple are buried, many believe they rest together in a Parisian cemetery where lovers and the lovelorn still visit to leave hopeful notes and messages to this day.

Bed

Sleeping alone in a double bed is sad luxury that I have become accustomed to. When, occasionally, I've had to sleep in a single bed I've been quite amazed that I didn't fall out of it during the night. Long ago I was very happy to share single beds with girlfriends; when you're young and in love, life is simple.

Sex Therapy

A few years ago, I went to see a sex therapist. I think that most of her clients were sex addicts, or couples with sexual problems in their relationships. I had quite a few appointments with her, and they weren't cheap, but I don't think there was really ever much she could have done to help me at all. She considered body language to be very important and encouraged me to acquire a more assertive demeanour so that I could come across as confident and make a more favourable impression on other people, particularly women. She also said that I was "stuck" and "resistant", which are not good things to be.

Lifespan

A couple of studies are occasionally cited as suggesting that eunuchs live longer than normal males.

One study conducted by Inha University in Incheon, South Korea, published in 2012, studied official records which covered three hundred years of the Imperial Korean court. In it, it was shown that 81 Korean eunuchs were found to have had an average life of seventy years and non-castrated men of the corresponding time had an average life expectancy in their fifties.

Another study published in 1969 by Hamilton and Mestler looked at the statistics of long-term inmates of a Kansas mental institution and found a similar variation between castrates and intact males. In the early part of the twentieth century it was a common practice to neuter some inmates of mental institutions.

It seems to be a theory, accepted by some, that castrating animals such as dogs, cats, and horses lengthens the lifespan of these animals.

It's possible that testosterone may account for a decreased life expectancy, as it's thought to suppress the immune system. Others suggest that increased levels of the hormone drive risky and aggressive behaviour.

Touch

I have lived as a recluse in plain sight, a castaway in the crowd. I am closed off in my personal darkness, yet long to open out and let the light in. I am untouched, an untouchable longing to be touched. Isolated, physically and emotionally, I crave intimacy – yet fear it too.

Young Love

A couple sit upon the grass in Whitworth Park on a summer day. They talk softly to each other, hands rest upon the other's thigh, they stroke each other's neck and hair. Gradually their faces converge, very slowly. Eventually their lips meet and begin the longest, slowest kiss. Time melts in the sunlight as they fuse together blissfully.

Letters

I used to write letters regularly to people I knew. As time has passed, and the internet has smothered the old ways, it is something done less often these days. What makes letter writing an archaic means of communication is exactly what makes it worth persevering with. It is personal; handwriting is individual, each person's containing distinctive, perhaps even peculiar, characteristics. It is slow; in a time-poor culture, making time for someone is a gesture that will be appreciated by them. It is as tactile an exchange as is possible remotely – the writer's hand has touched the paper and left their mark upon it for the one who will receive and hold it. Paper and skin – a vicarious contact; the paper or card that is chosen can itself express much too. Letters are suited to more profound exchanges, and even those that initially appear trivial might reveal much and say a great deal.

Torment

In Ancient Greek mythology, Tantalus was consigned to the lowest and darkest part of the underworld to endure an eternal punishment; he was forced to stand up to his neck in a cool pool of water, with succulent fruits hanging from the branches of trees just above his head. He was condemned to feel terrible hunger and be parched with thirst, but if he stretched a hand up towards the fruit the branches would move out of his reach. Likewise, if he stooped to drink the water, the level would immediately drop beyond him.

Beautiful women are my punishment. It twists me up inside to see them and know that I am not a man. I can walk around town and see any number of gorgeous women, each one a reminder of my wretchedness. Without any outlet for feelings that are constantly aroused within me I have become a psychologically deformed mutant, trapped in a disfigured condition. At least it will not be for eternity; that's something to be thankful for I suppose.

Origen

He was an early Christian theologian who wrote extensively and was an ascetic. He is said to have castrated himself in renunciation of physical pleasures. He was very influential but had many detractors who disagreed with some of his ideas, particularly those relating to the pre-existence of souls. He was later formally anathematised by the church. Self-castration was largely eradicated within the Catholic Church from the fifth century onwards.

Food

I am a rather boring person. I don't smoke cigarettes, drink alcohol, use drugs or gamble, and I've long forgotten what sex is like. Every loser needs at least one addiction, however – mine is unhealthy food. Eating gives me a false sense of comfort when I want to distract myself from uncomfortable feelings. In addition to eating the wrong sort of food, I also eat too much of it as well. Apparently, Casanova transformed into an obese librarian once he'd become impotent.

Food is the one sensual "pleasure" that I get to indulge in. It's not a pleasure, though, it's a compulsion that has inhibited my potential to have a happy life. Even though I'm not hungry, I shovel food into my mouth – bloating dulls the uncomfortable emotions that flare up regularly. Sometimes when I feel unhappy and tormented, I find myself opening the fridge to see what I can eat, or I pop out to the local shop to acquire some desperately needed chocolate. I gorge, then feel disgust and contempt for myself for being captive to this pathetic pattern.

Who Will Turn You Back?

When you are standing close to the edge, who will talk to you and prevent you going over? What if you look around, and there is no-one there? You are completely alone. The only person who can help now is the same one that has brought you here – yourself. Do not listen to the darkness, that is not really you; it is a shadow cast by disturbances of the light. You must listen to your true self, but first, you must find out who that is. Take time to do this please; it's very important that you do.

What Are You Reading?

When I see someone reading a book; in a coffee shop, or on a bench in the park, I often feel an urge to approach them and ask how the book makes them feel, and whether they would recommend it to someone else. Of course, I do no such thing, as most people wouldn't welcome such an impertinent enquiry from an old misfit.

In a Summer Garden

It's just a dream. The man walks through a dark cool room, then through wide French windows with delicate curtains swaying gently in the breeze. He steps out into the sunshine, stopping for a few seconds to get used to the light and heat. The paving stones burn gently, but once he's descended the steps the grass feels pleasant beneath his bare feet. He carefully carries a tray that has chilled glasses and a jug of ice-cubed deliciousness upon it. A line of trees ruffle, insects drone over vivid colours, the air shimmers blissfully. She is at the far end, near the bloom-covered wall, reclining comfortably on the bench. Cushions have been brought out from the house, as well as a table; she wears a wide-brimmed straw hat and reads her book. He stops for a moment, admiring her discreetly. When he lays the tray upon the table, she smiles at him, he fills the two glasses and she puts the book down – once she has marked her place in it. She sits upright for a moment as he settles beside her, then leans back against him after removing her hat. He wraps an arm around her waist, and she holds his wrist. The juice tastes good. He rests his chin on the top of her head, and she sighs softly. They share a perfect silence; there is nothing to be said.

Reviews

I enjoy reading book reviews in the weekend papers. It's much easier sometimes to just read a review about a book rather than having to plough through the book itself. Often a review is more interesting than the book in question, anyhow. I'm a slow reader; it takes me a while to work my way through a lot of pages, especially if the prose is the sort where you have to keep going back so you can try to understand what you've just read. So, it makes sense to read the reviews instead. Often an approving appraisal has tempted me into buying the book, but in many cases I haven't got around to actually reading it yet, and there's a chance I never will either. Reviews can provoke an emotional response by themselves; be informative and influence opinions just as much as any book, if not more sometimes.

The First Time

One evening, my dad was working a late shift, and there was just me and Mum watching the old black and white television set that we had. A programme came on that featured a couple of piano players; many years later I realised that the show consisted of two separate performances spliced together. I watched the screen in a puzzled state of excitement – it was my first encounter with rock'n'roll. The performers were Little Richard and Jerry Lee Lewis. Both had backing bands and an audience that responded to the music with uninhibited joy. I recall Little Richard taking his jacket off and his shirt being drenched with sweat. When Jerry Lee played, some of the audience were arranged on a scaffolding stage set, but soon a frantic mob crowded around the piano as they became possessed by the music.

Hijra

In several south Asian countries, there are people who are sometimes officially recognised as being of a third sex. The hijras of India, Pakistan, Bangladesh and Sri Lanka are usually transsexual, but not all are castrated. There are many complex aspects to Hijra culture, which has been in existence for many centuries – they're mentioned in the *Kama Sutra*. Some hijras undergo the removal of genitalia as part of a ritual lasting several days. They live in tightly knit communities and are social outcasts, generally despised by the majority of the population. Many speak a secret language, called Hijra Farsi or Koti, which is known only to members of their community. During previous centuries they had held a comparatively respected place in society, but under the British Raj suffered brutal persecution and continue to experience prejudice to this day. They scrape a living from sex work, begging and performing at functions. The eunuch's curse is considered by some to be a terrible misfortune, whilst their blessing is thought auspicious. The power of both of these is believed particularly potent in relation to life-cycle events – marriage and children, sex and love. It is thought that as hijras have no outlet for their own sexual energy, the accumulation of this gives them the power to bestow a boon or a bane upon others. Hijras perform at weddings and other occasions, such as birth events and birthday celebrations, dancing and singing for *badhai* – gifts of cash and goods that include sweets, cloth and grains.

In Bihar province the authorities employed hijras to help recover unpaid municipal taxes from defaulting shopkeepers and business owners. A group of twenty garishly dressed performers would sing and dance outside appropriate premises, often encouraging prompt payments to be made to the accompanying revenue official by embarrassed debtors. They are also employed as security guards in women's refuges, as they will not sexually assault or harass the female inmates staying there.

The most recent census in India recorded half a million transgender individuals, but it is thought that this total is greater in reality as there's a deep stigma attached to a group who have existed on the margins of society for centuries.

The Ramayana is an ancient Indian epic poem estimated to have been composed two and a half thousand years ago. It narrates the struggle of the divine prince Rama against the demon King Ravana to free his beloved wife Sita. In some versions of this tale Rama leaves to enter the forest and is followed by many of his subjects; Rama stops and addresses them. He instructs them not to mourn his departure and commands all men and women of his kingdom to return to the city. Fourteen years later, he returned to discover that a group of eunuchs had remained at the place where he had given his speech, and as they were neither men nor women they had stayed there, awaiting his return. Rama was touched by their devotion and granted them the power to confer blessings at inaugural occasions such as births and marriages.

South Indian hijras sometimes refer to themselves as Aravanis. This relates to the story from the Mahabharat, an epic Indian legend, where Aravan promises to give his life in battle the following day but asks Shiva if he can marry before dying. No woman will have him, so Shiva assumes the form of a very beautiful woman called Mohini and becomes his wife for a single night. Hijras claim to be the product of this coupling.

Imperfectly Perfect

When a guitar is in tune it's good to play, but if all the strings are *exactly* in tune, it's just too much. If there is a barely perceptible, slightly off-centre pitch to a string or two then it is wonderfully perfect to make music with.

Memory

It seems that every time we remember something, our brain creates new neurones and the synaptic connections are altered. Effectively, we do not remember an event, but actually remember the last time we remembered it. Each time we access a memory it becomes altered by the act of recollection. Perhaps emotional and psychological perspectives can also influence this process; we all have a selective memory at times, don't we? Perhaps our memories are *not* who we are, or think we are. Our self-knowledge is often built upon questionable foundations.

Crying

Men who have been treated with androgen deprivation therapy often report an increased tendency to being moody and emotional. I would concur with that; when I've had low testosterone levels, I've found myself becoming quite sentimental and sensitive, with an increased tendency to tearfulness.

Professor Richard Wassenburg was diagnosed and treated for prostate cancer; he underwent androgen deprivation therapy – sometimes known as "chemical castration". He has written some interesting pieces and noted that his altered hormonal status led to his memory becoming less reliable, his muscle turning into fat, and his body hair disappearing. He also indicated a frequent inclination to cry – "since my castration I'll weep at road safety commercials". He obviously still kept his sense of humour. Richard explained that he feared his more frequent tearfulness might be construed as maudlin self-pity but realised that he had just become more sensitive to other people. He suggested that his experience had led him to believe that testosterone suppresses empathy and fuels aggression.

Killing Our Mother

We are poisoning the Earth with toxic pollution, yet sneer at previous generations in history for their ignorance and hypocrisy. In the future, people will look back upon us and our time and despise us for our selfishness in bequeathing a poisoned planet to them. They will condemn us for ignoring uncomfortable truths, and curse us for our greed. But so what – it won't be our problem, will it?

Libido and Sex Drive

These two terms often seem to be used interchangeably, but from my experience I would suggest that they might be considered as two separate entities. Sometimes, when

I was using an older type of testosterone injection, I would experience episodes when I had relentless erections – even though I wasn't in the slightest turned on or aroused emotionally. It was as if my body was primed for sex, but I wasn't. This led me to think of sex drive as being the physical readiness and ability to act or perform sexually. Libido, on the other hand, is more about what you feel emotionally and what you're thinking – a psychological arousal. I noted an occasional displacement between the two; when I was going through one of the spells when my body was geared up, my emotions didn't match up with my body at first, but would be drawn along behind it with a slight delay. After a few days my physical sex drive began to drop back to normal levels, but my thoughts and feelings were still greatly aroused for a while after, before receding once more. I found it to be particularly difficult when my emotions were pumped up, my psyche inflamed, but my body was no longer part of the circus. I can also say from experience that being horny all the time is quite a miserable state to be in, too; you are enslaved by sexual desire – it's really not much fun being like that.

Synthetic Masculinity

Testosterone, along with other hormones, was synthesised in 1935 by two biochemists working separately – Leopold Ruzicka and Adolf Butenandt. They were awarded the Nobel Prize for Chemistry jointly in 1939.

What We Really Want

That's what consumer capitalism gives us, only we don't know what we want until it tells us. Things – houses, cars, consumer goods. Experiences – holidays and entertainments. Emotions – rage, resentment, and contempt. Let's not forget alienation and depression either. Hoorah for the global free market!

Beautiful Mediocrity

How would I know the difference between a virtuoso and a mediocrity? I'd need a qualified expert to tell me which was which a lot of the time. Yet, if I listen or observe with my heart, it is often the "lesser" performer that leaves the technically adept behind. You can discern the *reason* behind a performance if you try; the "why" of it. All that is done in love is done well. By this process, base material can be conjured into the most precious and beautiful of elements. But, you have to remember how to be aware of this, a power that we forget we have because of learnt opinions and conditioned perceptions. If any art becomes a collection of dextrous showpieces and dazzling techniques, it loses its magic. Yet stumbling ineptitude can express a deep and wonderful sense of soul that will often elude those more capable. Sometimes those who do something badly do it much better than those who do it well.

Zombie

For many years, I was little more than a walking corpse. I existed and interacted with people around me in a seemingly normal way, but this was only a performance that deceived myself as much as anyone else. Inside, behind the mask that I thought was my face, my spirit was shrivelled and desiccated. I had shut down and allowed a myth to be written in my heart that cursed me with a false identity; it was just a self-pitying lie. I recited destructive chants everyday internally, hateful monologues that reminded me of my worthlessness. The rage was never released, but contained within me, I nurtured it by feeding it resentment and shame. I was consumed in toxic flames, and each day rose like a poisoned phoenix to admire myself in a distorted mirror of twisted perception where the more I hated myself, the more everything seemed solid and certain. It was a safe discomfort zone to exist in, where I was unchallenged, where I did not have to face up to fear...or myself.

The Seasons

When I was young, I didn't pay much attention to the seasons. Now I have lived through over a half-century of annual cycles, I look out for the little changes that mark the passing of time; the anticipation of things to come, the short-lived memory of things recently past. I bore people by informing them of the approaching solstice or equinox, or tell them to look out for a perigee moon that always underwhelms them when they see it in the sky.

Andy Warhol

I didn't think much of him until I read some of his books; then I was a bit more impressed. His superficiality concealed a deep understanding of how western culture works and some of the less noble aspects of human nature. He was very quotable; here are a couple of observations –

"Sex is the biggest nothing of all time."

"The most exciting thing is not doing it; if you fall in love with someone and never do it, it's more exciting."

Sunshine Girl

Adolescent summers included occasional visits to a farm, where one of the daughters sat in a wild garden, whiling away slow afternoons with her friends. One particularly caught my attention, inspiring the most innocent desire; a girl with sun-burnished legs and a golden bob. She read beneath the sun, coolly indifferent to my amazement at her, brushing off clumsy attempts at conversation.

A year or two later I had stretched into another body, my voice deepening. Overheard grown-up conversations mentioned an accident, a car driven by one of the local tearaways – no legal requirement to wear seatbelts back then. A further visit on a rainy day, tea and biscuits in a front room. She was there, subdued and pale, assurance gone. A mirror above the fireplace permitted discreet observation whilst adults exchanged dreariness. A couple of times I looked up and caught her regarding me in the glass, her eyes quickly turned away, but I saw. She was looking at *me*! I still smile in disbelief decades later.

I wish I could have told her, that last time I saw her, the scars on her face made no difference. She was still, just… beautiful. She always will be.

Zuihitsu

It's usually taken to mean "follow the brush" – a genre of Japanese literature that consists of loosely connected personal observations, fragmented ideas and reflections, miscellaneous musings, insights and observations. These are all woven together to compose an unplanned collected whole, where the text might "drift like a cloud", becoming a random scrapbook that may tell many stories by telling no story at all.

Radio Four

I listen to this station regularly and find myself randomly tuned into unexpected and interesting reflections and ideas. Often, I despair about our culture and the direction that it is taking, but when I listen to BBC Radio 4, I am reassured that civilised discussion, respectful behaviour, and tolerant values may still be found in our country.

Writer-ish

It is a language that I have tried to learn without much success. I express myself in clichés, employ excessive adjectives, and have a very basic grasp of punctuation.

But I've got something to say, and I'm darned well going to say it…even if I don't really know what it is that I want to tell you.

Young Love

In North Tea Power, a boy and girl discuss what to get for their kitchen. They've been shopping for household items to go in their new place, having just moved in together. They share coffee, breathless excitement, and a sweet hopefulness. Just like newly-weds I think – beautifully unblemished and strong, unsullied by defeat, pure and uncomplicated in their joy. I silently bestow a eunuch's blessing upon them and wish them much happiness in the future. I hope that they will choose some nice crockery too.

Self Esteem

Having a low level of self-esteem may not be a road to happiness, but I'd also have to say that a lot of harmful and dangerous people seem to have an unreasonably inflated opinion of themselves and their capabilities. Those with high self-esteem often seem to be the ones that cause most of the damage in the world, whilst those with low self-esteem may only inhibit opportunities for their own happiness.

I think that self-respect is an entirely different matter from self-esteem, but both are often confused with each other. Those who respect themselves will also respect other people and the world around them, whilst those with little self-respect will often inflict harm upon others as a result of this.

Please Like Me

I really wanted people to like me. I sought other people's approval and tried to buy it by giving them things – objects or attention. I thought that if I was useful to them then they would like me more; I was desperate for their approval because I didn't value myself. I didn't realise that this was the case until I fell into the abyss, and my self-deluding constructions of identity were stripped away. People see through supplicatory gestures quickly, and regard such a need for affirmation with justified disdain. It's natural to want other people to like you, but it's unhealthy to allow this desire to become the major motivation for your actions. You are only chasing an un-catchable rainbow if you do.

Good Film Endings Without Dialogue

The final scene of *The Third Man*; the tiresomely righteous good guy is completely blanked by the girl who loved the bad guy that sold her down the river.

In *Fat City*, the two men have nothing to say to each other, but drink coffee together. The younger one stays so that the old, broken one will not be alone.

In *Broadway Danny Rose*, he runs out onto the street after the woman who screwed him over comes to say sorry – a beautiful act of forgiveness.

In *Cinema Paradiso*, Toto watches the montage of cut scenes that Alfredo has left for him. They are the screen kisses and romantic embraces that were censored by the local priest over many years.

The Arndale

I used to dislike visiting the Arndale; I snobbishly regarded it as a temple to soulless consumerism. Maybe I've lightened up a bit, but I quite like having a stroll around there now. Sometimes I imagine it like the scene from *The Fisher King*, where all the commuters in the railway station dance together. Unlike the film, I never spot the special woman in the crowd, but maybe one day?

Note to Self

You're useless! You can't even do the most basic things without messing them up. You're a complete waste of space, you fat crap. Look at yourself, what a worthless lump of rubbish you turned out to be.

Zheng He

He's considered to be one of China's great explorers. Taken prisoner by Ming soldiers in 1381, he was castrated shortly afterwards. He served in the court of a Chinese prince and commanded forces in a successful rebellion against the reigning emperor. He acquired great power once his master had taken the throne. He is famous in China for the expeditions he led throughout the Indian Ocean to South Asia and East Africa that opened up new routes for trade. These voyages were undertaken by a great fleet of ships which included the world's largest vessels of the day.

Plasticity

Men don't really know what they want, but whatever it may be – they *really* want it. And, women have it. Male desire is a relentlessly powerful force that is also very suggestible. Women are the eternal objects of male preoccupation and are themselves often shaped by the passions of men, so that they assume forms that they are culturally moulded into – physically and otherwise. In some past societies, small feet were prized, and consequently young girls had their feet bound to prevent them growing. In others a long neck was considered an ideal of feminine beauty, and girls had rings placed around their necks to lengthen them unnaturally. In our culture, women have plastic surgery to acquire features that conform to a plastic ideal of female desirability and beauty. But, just as women are moulded to conform to what is thought to be a male idea of sexual perfection, the desires of men are also malleable. Their fantasies are formed by social conditioning, and the insidious power of suggestion too. The forces that shape perceptions are adjustable and controllable; our entertainments, media, and advertising send out a continuous stream of subliminal messages which influence thoughts and behaviour.

Dazlious

Comic book word scrabble is a game played by Sigourney Weaver and Alan Rickman in the film *Snowcake*. Made-up words are permissible but must be used in a sentence by the players submitting them. There's a clip of it on YouTube that I like to watch sometimes. Alan

Rickman's character (Alex) asks Sigourney Weaver's (Linda) for an example of the word she has just placed upon the board.

She responds – "Mister Fantastic, from the Fantastic Four, he's got arms made of elastic so they can stretch for two, maybe three hundred miles. He's been imprisoned in a cave for seven days with no food and no water and no light. On the eighth day he manages to loosen a rock and push his way up through the top and up into the daylight, just as the sun is coming up over the mountains and filling the sky with this white-yellow light. And there's a stillness, and in the few minutes he's got before his captor, the evil Doctor Doom, returns, he stops for one second. And all he can hear is his own breathing, and he's totally overwhelmed by how big the world is, and how small and unimportant he is. And as he turns around you see his face look to the sky and he says very quietly, so that no-one can hear him, he says – 'dazlious'." Near the end of the film, Alex uses this made-up word to express wonderment.

The Last Handwritten Newspaper in the World

The Musulman is a daily evening paper that is printed in Chennai. It's written in Urdu, a minority language in that city, and is a tiny operation kept afloat by having just enough subscribers to ensure its continuing survival. Three calligraphers and a couple of reporters are employed on modest pay, all of them believe passionately in the project. The masthead and advertisements are, literally, cut and pasted onto a blank sheet, then the columns are marked out and the calligraphers begin to produce their magic. All involved with this enterprise deeply love the language itself and are resolved to continue their endeavours in the face of an ever-precarious future.

Etymology

The name is often a pejorative one. Its origin lies in ancient Greek; one theory is it meant "guarding the bed", whilst another opinion is that its original meaning was "being good with respect to the mind". The term "eunuch" is normally used to describe men who have been physically castrated. Some suggest the name has also in the past been applied to those who abstain from sex, are homosexual or transgender. There has been discussion whether women who have had their reproductive organs removed might also come under this description, but the term never seems to be applied to them. Those who have undergone female genital mutilation, sometimes described as female circumcision, are perhaps also comparable to male eunuchs, even though reproductive capability may remain unaltered.

The Other Half

In Plato's *Symposium,* the myth of the other half is laid out by Aristophanes. Once upon a time, human beings had four legs, four arms and two faces. The immortals were wary of these beings and Zeus, the ruler of the gods, decided to cut each human being in half to diminish their power. The humans longed deeply for their lost other half and searched the world for them; if two halves discovered each other they wrapped themselves in an embrace and would not let go – "the pair are lost in an amazement of love and friendship and intimacy".

In the myth, the children of the sun were male, and the children of the earth were female, whilst the children of the moon were a third sex that had both male and female elements. Perhaps some people are distorted – incomplete pieces that have no complementary other half that might fit with them. They are condemned to wander the earth, consumed by loneliness, and dream about what cannot ever be.

Having a Crush

It is a way of experiencing attraction to someone else, and the emotions associated with this, without reality being allowed to intrude and spoil everything. There is no wish to express or act upon the feelings; it is a safe, displaced attachment that is classically associated with young teenage girls. They will grow up into young women, will move on – but I am stuck in a retarded state. It is not healthy for an old eunuch to have a crush on younger women; many would say it's quite creepy. It is a symptom of a deformed emotional condition, a retrograde immaturity acquired by my lostness.

Over the years I've had secret admirations for a few women, but it really had little to do with them in the slightest. It was all about unexpressed impulses that were trapped within my damaged psyche. I didn't try to make anything happen or nurture any hopes that it might. Thankfully, I never expressed these feelings to anyone except you, otherwise I really would have embarrassed myself. The women who I had these secret attachments to represented something that was lost to me, something I wanted but could never have.

Three Rules of Our Culture

1. Greed is good
2. Look after Number One
3. There is no such thing as "society"

Wicked

A woman wants to experience emotions when she's with a man, and a "bad guy" will provoke a lot more feelings than a dull, "nice boy" ever could. She'll be swept up by the passions he arouses within her, even though she probably realises that there will be a price to pay later. It's like a night on the town; after a couple of tequilas she feels *really* good and is in the mood for an absolute blow-out. She knows that in the morning she'll be ill, kneeling on the floor whilst throwing up into the toilet. But, so what? Let tomorrow take care of itself, tonight she's going to have fun. She will dance on tables, laugh and sing, and feel so intoxicatingly, exuberantly...alive! Douchebags are like tequila; they possess a powerful kick of excitement that comes with dangerous after-effects. Respectful, caring men are like low-calorie fruit juice; perhaps it's healthy but it's so boring! Girls just wanna have fun, and why not? Even the bad-boy hangover is more stimulating than anything that a dreary loser can offer. The dangerous guy possesses a far larger palette of exciting colours than the small range of insipid paleness offered by the safe and reliable drip. Compare a vibrantly messy, oil-spattered canvas and an insignificantly drab water colour – guess which one provokes the more powerful response. Would the lady prefer a ride on a roller-coaster, or a mobility scooter? Mm, that's a tough one.

A woman may care for a man who is kind and loving,

but she will also vainly wish that he could excite and arouse her too. He doesn't, because he can't, and never will. She may come to have contempt for him because he cannot make her feel like a complete woman. She might wish that this wasn't true, but not be able to conjure emotions by an effort of will, no matter how hard she may try. She cannot choose what turns her on; unsummoned desires arise within her no matter how she tries to suppress them – they are too strong. She can't help herself. Bad guys are more fun in bed, they're creative and funny, they make things happen. Bad is *so* delicious… and irresistible… and fun.

Remaining Afloat

When a large ship is holed below the waterline, disaster may be avoided by prompt action. Doors are closed and hatches secured. The breach will be contained within a section enclosed by watertight compartments which are integral to the vessel's structure. The ship will remain afloat, even though parts of it are flooded.

I didn't sink. My boat sat low in the water, the steering and engines damaged, but at least it remained afloat. I sailed in a wide circle upon the ocean's surface and convinced myself that I was travelling towards a destination somewhere. I was on a voyage to nowhere, using a defective compass and the wrong charts.

After too long I realised that I must put into dry dock for essential repairs; I must somehow find a port. There has been extensive internal corrosion, leaks are becoming increasingly apparent, sealed compartments are no longer watertight. A complete refit is required – perhaps I've left it too late.

Approaching the City

Years ago, I would come into the city by train; my heart would quicken with anticipation as the carriages drew nearer to the tall towers of the centre. Sometimes the destination was Victoria, and I'd peer through smudged glass as gleaming buildings glided by. Sometimes the train passed through Oxford Road on its way to Piccadilly, and I would look down upon grubby streets full of possibilities as we became absorbed into the body of the city.

These days I drive into the city, have done so countless times, yet always feel a shiver of excitement when the ziggurats first reveal themselves briefly as the road crests a hill. Recollections flicker of childhood excursions to the beach; we'd search the shifting horizon for the moment of promise which would cause great excitement – "Look, the sea!" A shimmering of unknown possibilities is waiting.

A Private Place

Even that most personal space in my psyche isn't mine. I never had a room of my own, no truly private place to be myself. My most secret thoughts and fantasies have always had an overbearing presence, a disapproving critic that I'm continually forced to justify myself to. For too long I felt guilt about having normal human feelings and have constantly squirmed under the interrogation of a bully calling itself my conscience. I have slowly tried to free myself, to start again new, but it's difficult.

Teaching Yourself

Often you will read something, and a light of recognition will glow inside you when someone expresses something that you had sensed inside yourself, but not been able to formulate into an explicit thought. I have found that this also happens when you write – you put something down on paper that you've snatched from somewhere in your head and look unbelievingly at what you've written. Where did it come from? You've taught yourself something that you already knew but hadn't realised.

The Big Water

There is only one body of water on Earth; all the lakes, rivers and seas are constituents of this, as are the clouds, rain, snow and ice. This single element may seem to be dispersed into many separate entities at any particular instant in a continuous state of flux, but they are all one. It may evaporate, and freeze; its location and state may alter, but these are only transient conditions of existence.

It has been said we are raindrops falling upon the ocean, and that when the drop meets the sea it becomes the ocean – but, it is also said by some that when this happens, it is actually the ocean that becomes the drop.

Not Giving a Fuck

It's the ultimate badge of honour in our culture. The less someone cares about others, and other people's feelings and opinions, the greater affirmation of individual worth it is. As social cohesion breaks down, we can expect very painful and poisonous times ahead whilst all drowning together in a toxic sea of contempt.

Saint Peter's Square

It's changed quite a bit over time. I remember years ago that there was a music shop where the Number One building now stands. I once got into a chat there with the owner about Cliff Gallup and early rock'n'roll. Nowadays, it's a pedestrianised piazza with tram stops, benches, and streams of people ceaselessly coming and going. Recently, a chap has started playing a saxophone near the water feature on Fridays, he plays a string of long slow notes, which occasionally resemble a melody you might have heard once somewhere. It's a place where people meet. I like watching someone waiting for their girlfriend or boyfriend and seeing their face light up with a smile when they arrive. A kiss on the cheek, a brief exchange of words, then the couple stroll towards the restaurant, or theatre, or wherever it is that they're going. Sometimes I imagine that I'm waiting there for someone special, and she's really late. It seems like I've been waiting for years; decades even. Finally, I see her approaching; she raises her hand in a casual wave and smiles, and my heart leaps inside me. I know then that everything is going to be alright after all.

Learning to Swim the Hard Way

I clung on to my pain desperately. In dangerous waters, a concrete life jacket seemed a solid and safe thing to hold tightly to, a necessary piece of equipment for survival. It kept pulling me under and I continuously struggled towards the surface to avoid drowning. Eventually I let go of my dangerous delusion, or was it torn away from me? I was saved by defeat; I had resisted rescue for so long.

Liu Jin

Leader of The Eight Tigers, a powerful group of eunuchs during the Ming dynasty that effectively controlled the imperial court, Liu Jin is regarded as being one of the most corrupt officials in Chinese history. He appropriated vast wealth and was implicated in a plot to overthrow the Emperor and was condemned to "death by a thousand cuts" – a lengthy process of torture and execution where a knife was used to methodically remove portions of the body over an extended period of time, eventually resulting in death. He suffered a particularly slow and agonising demise, remaining alive for an unusually long time whilst the sentence was being carried out.

Sylvia Potts

I can still recall the effect that the race had; the ending was replayed on the television repeatedly for a few days, and then I only had my memories of it for over forty years until someone uploaded a clip to YouTube with inappropriately mocking music. How many winners and medallists have I watched triumphantly crossing finishing lines since then? Yet it is a woman that finished ninth in the 1500m women's final of the 1970 Commonwealth Games that has left the most powerful impression upon me – I will probably never forget it as long as I live. Her name was Sylvia Potts. She wore the all-black kit of New Zealand as she came around the final bend and accelerated into the home straight. Rita Ridley, of England, came with her as they moved ahead of the field. Photographs of those final moments show the suffering upon the faces of all the runners as they summon up every last vestige of effort from the deepest core of their being. Sylvia was in front going into the last few strides of the race, then her body seized up, her legs would not work anymore. She fell to the ground agonisingly short of the line with a painfully ungraceful crash. Her body had nothing left to give. Rita herself has barely the energy to lift her arms as her momentum carries her to a surprise victory, other runners pass the crumpled athlete as she realises what has happened. Her instincts compel her to get to her feet; it is a great struggle to do this, but she succeeds. She can barely stand; she sucks in desperate lungfuls of air then unsteadily staggers over the line somehow.

Sylvia represented New Zealand at an Olympics and two Commonwealth Games; she made the semi-finals of the 1968 Olympics and came fifth in the 800m final of the 1970 Commonwealth Games. Nobody can give more than everything that they have, and one wet day in Edinburgh long ago that's exactly what Sylvia Potts did. That is why she will always be one of the greatest runners I've ever seen.

The Galli of Ancient Greece and Rome

Cybele was a mother goddess who was revered by the people of Phrygia, a place that now lies within modern Turkey. Her consort was Attis, a god of vegetation, whose emasculation, death and resurrection were said to represent the fruits of the earth that die in winter, only to be reborn in spring. Reverence for Cybele and Attis was transferred from Greece to Rome; the priests who devoted themselves to these deities were eunuchs, known as Galli. They castrated themselves in an ecstatic celebration that was held every March 24th, known as The Day of Blood. Those Galli, who were already eunuchs, would cut or flog themselves until they bled and danced rapturously whilst dressed in yellow.

Biblical Eunuchs

"No-one who is emasculated by cutting or crushing may enter the assembly of the Lord." – Deuteronomy xxii, 1

"Let no eunuch say – 'Behold, I am only a dried-up tree'. For thus says the Lord – 'To the eunuchs who keep my Sabbaths, who choose what pleases me and hold fast my covenant. To them I will give, within my house and its walls, a memorial and a name far better than sons and daughters could give. I will give each of them an everlasting name that will never be cut off'." – Isaiah lvi, 3

"There are eunuchs born that way, there are eunuchs made that way by men, and there are those who have made themselves eunuchs for the kingdom of heaven. The one who can accept it should accept it."– Matthew ixx, 12

Note to Self

Who'd want you? You've got the charisma and personality of a puddle; you've nothing interesting to say whatsoever. You look disgusting, a big bloated blob of blubber. You're just an impotent, sterile eunuch.

Confined Reading

In my dark and desolate years, when I languished in a jail within my head, I read books by those who had been imprisoned by cruel regimes. Their inspiring stories emphasised to me how strong some people could be when faced with impossible situations. Their books are powerful and inspiring, if sometimes difficult, reading.

Life and Death in Shanghai, by Nien Cheng
Man's Search for Meaning, by Viktor Frankl
If This is a Man – The Truce, by Primo Levi
Grey is the Colour of Hope, by Irina Ratushinskaya
A Day in the Life of Ivan Denisovich, by Alexander Solzenitsyn
Night, by Elie Weisel

Shrivelled Fruit

Love is for young people. Bodies degrade when they get older, and decline is not just physical – hearts lose their sweetness as they wither with age.

Internet Dating

I was a member of a well-known dating site for several years in total, but never actually got a date out of it. I spent a fair amount of money on membership subscriptions, and wasted many hours looking hopefully for a nice woman, but all in vain. At first, I would spend an evening sifting through ladies' profiles and after much consideration decide upon the one who seemed the most suitable. I'd send her a message, and then wait for a reply that never came. Eventually I learnt that it's a numbers game and that it's advisable to cast a wide net, to contact a large number of women and see what results. This seemed rather an indiscriminate approach, and I still didn't get much interest when I tried it. I was looking for a woman who was up to five years older or younger than me but noted that most women indicated a preference for men significantly younger than themselves. It seems that a lot of men are seeking younger women too, so I don't know how it all adds up in reality. A few times I'd get into a brief exchange of messages with ladies via the site, but this always fizzled out to nothing. I was contacted by a few fake profiles; there are many scams aiming to snare hopeful hearts. I made many changes to my profile in an attempt to find the magic formula, but I never struck gold, not even the fool's variety. I think internet dating can be good for attractive and confident people, as well as those seeking no-strings fun, but might be less useful for those who aren't so appealing and hoping for a more committed relationship with someone. The companies that run dating websites are only interested in profits and those seeking love are easy prey.

Pollution

Our emotional environment has become toxic; we inhale and ingest psychological poisons continuously. Micro-aggressions accumulate within us, causing us to be increasingly alienated from each other and more furious at each other. We then fill ourselves up with even more poison, in the mistaken belief that it is a medicine that will cure us of the chronic conditions that destroy us from the inside, but we only end up make ourselves sicker. The first step to getting clean is to stop being angry, but it is the hardest step of all to take. It is also the most important one.

The Magical Time

I think many bands are at their most potent when they've been together from a few months until about a year or so. After that, they can still be very good in some ways, but they'll have lost something special by no longer being inchoate and reaching towards places they weren't sure existed within themselves. It takes a little while for a band to find itself and pull together, but that anything-could-happen period where they are uncertain of what they are, or what they are trying to be, is often when they are at their most unknowingly beautiful. Many collapse when the pieces don't fit together, or become lost in confusion, but some touch an elusive wonderful without knowing how they did it, or even that they have done it at all. This phenomenon contains many variables that are dependent upon the talents and abilities of those involved, their attitude and aspirations, and pure chance. Once a band has settled upon a firm formula to work with, they start losing the unpredictable and chaotic magic that they possessed during their earlier enchanted dreamtime.

Hidden Terror

Some psychologists suggest that a woman's deepest fear when she meets a new man is that he will cause her physical harm, whilst a man's deepest fear when he begins interacting with a woman is that she will humiliate him sexually. Men are terrified of having their manliness belittled by women; perhaps such a fear caused me to subconsciously sabotage my chances of having what I wanted more than anything else – a loving relationship with a good woman. I can't tell you how much I despise myself now that I realise that this might have been the case.

Coming Out Jealousy

It is a very good thing that people can be more honest about themselves these days, and that other people are prepared to accept those who don't conform to old, restrictive identities. In recent years, there have been a few chaps that play traditionally "macho" sports, who have publicly revealed their sexuality, I hope that this helps other people and will also make our culture even more tolerant. I must also admit to feeling jealousy when I read about these men coming out as gay; whilst they were "living a lie" they had little trouble getting women to love them, marry them and have children together. They didn't really want a woman but seemed to have their pick of them, whilst I wanted a woman more than anything and couldn't get one. They may be gay, but they're men – which is more than I'll ever be.

Nobody's Daddy

When I was a young man, it was sometimes suggested that I would make a good father someday; I was caring, patient and kind. A girlfriend was late once and after nearly a fortnight said that, if she was pregnant, she would have the baby and we would be a family. She started her period soon after – we split up a few months later.

Vasily Arkhipov

On the 27th October 1962 American warships located a Soviet submarine near Cuba and began dropping depth charges as it submerged into deep waters. It transpired later that the US Navy had no inkling that the submarine was carrying a nuclear weapon, and that a heated discussion was taking place between senior officers below the surface. The submarine's captain, Valetin Savitsky, was adamant that the nuclear weapon should be deployed and was strongly supported by the political officer, Ivan Masslenikov. The command protocol for this particular submarine differed from the others in its flotilla in that the three senior officers onboard had to be unanimous in approving the use of the nuclear option; the other vessels only required the captain's order be supported by the political officer. The third officer that day on submarine B-59 was Vasily Arkhipov who, as flotilla commander, held equal rank with the captain. He had been on board submarine K-19 the previous year when a fault in its reactor had led to the entire crew being exposed to massive levels of radiation, causing many subsequent deaths. His courageous role in this event had led to him commanding great respect within the Soviet submarine service. Captain Arkhipov calmly reasoned that there was no evidence that war had broken out and that the submarine should surface and seek orders from Moscow. He eventually prevailed and the commencement of nuclear conflict was avoided. One of President Kennedy's advisors later described the incident as "the most dangerous in human history". When B-59 returned to base the crew were told by an admiral that it would have been better had they gone down with their ship and never returned. Olga, Arkhipov's wife, described him as intelligent, polite and calm, and said that he disliked speaking of the incident that remained largely unknown during his lifetime. It wasn't until 2002 that the occurrences of that day were publicised by a junior officer who had been on board. Vasily Arkhipov was a good and humble man who may well have saved the world from nuclear war.

Understanding

Knowing something in your heart is different from knowing it in your mind – the latter's like a 3D movie seen without the special spectacles, a stream of information without the encryption code. Wisdom of the heart is a most precious blessing.

Salford Sunflowers

They're building apartments there now. For a few years it was a wild pop-up meadow that in summer had waist-high daisies visited by butterflies and bees. Once there were sunflowers too; I planted and tended them over several months. I was inspired by a quote and a short story. The quote was from Anne Herbert; she said – "Practice random kindness and senseless acts of beauty". It was the second part of this that I tried to make real on some waste ground. There was also a Rudyard Kipling piece – 'Fairy-Kist' – an over-worded mystery that includes a gentle soul who had been damaged by the Great War. He planted flowers at night in unlikely locations, in response to the darkness that had broken his mind.

I grew them from seedlings in pots in a distant back-yard, then planted them in the meadow once they were strong enough to survive on their own. I permitted myself the use of compost, but not insecticide; the plants turned out to be very popular with slugs.

Herons were regular visitors to the canal lock beside the meadow. I'd never heard them calling to each other before – they'd always been silent birds to me. I saw hawks hover, and once one swooped and rose again with a mouse or shrew in its talons. Dog-walkers passed by whilst I scratched at the thin soil with forks and trowels. I made regular runs in the car, with watering cans in the back, ensuring the tall fragile stems would not dry out.

Cane and twine, hope and idiocy. A young couple were regular visitors. They'd promenade through the swaying grass and sit by the disused basin cross-legged, facing each other. The head of each slowly leaning forward towards the other; she demonstrative gestures, he gentle patience. I hope that they had a happy summer, and if they are still together, I would be really pleased about that too.

I planted dozens and nurtured them; I cannot be angry at the snails for eating them. Eventually, half a dozen bloomed for a few weeks with distant follies forming an angular backdrop to my temporary meadow. I'd like to think that someone passing may have stopped one day, spotting an incongruity, and thought to themselves – "sunflowers"?

Ly Thuong Kiet

He was a Vietnamese eunuch of the eleventh century who served in the Imperial Cavalry with distinction and was promoted to the rank of General. China blockaded its southern neighbour whilst preparing for an invasion but Ly Thuong Kiet led a pre-emptive attack across the border and the Chinese forces were defeated after extensive fighting. The following year a Chinese army combined with Khmer and Champa forces to invade Vietnam. Though outnumbered, Ly Thuong Kiet led a

resourceful defence that showed him to be a wily strate-
gist, and the invasion was defeated. He is still revered in
Vietnam and there is a shrine to him in Hanoi.

Some Obscure Treasures on 7" Vinyl

Wishing Well, by Glo-Worm (Slumberland) – A
band that existed for only a few weeks.
Chiming guitars and clattering percussion with
a mannered, soaring vocal on green vinyl.

Days Are Getting Shorter, by Poconos (Jigsaw) –
Boy/Girl duo with half a dozen songs on blue
vinyl. Breathless female and throwaway male
vocals with minimal instrumentation make this
a sweetly awkward pleasure.

The 13th Century, by Norfolk Rider (Dutch
Courage) – A delightful postal collaboration.
Two bands (Norfolk & Western and Shoes &
Rider) tape vocals and guitar and send to the
other for embellishment.

An Abstract of the Anti Anti-Folk Manifesto, by Ben
Hanisch (Intercontinental) – A Herman Dune
twin goes to the East Village on a French label
with touching results.

Sleepy & Sleeper, by Clean Boy*Messy Girl
(Clover) – From Tokyo on blue vinyl. The

wonderfully clumsy popsters get their acoustic
guitars out and charm your pants off.

In Search of the Radiant Sun, by Mohagonny
(Elefant) – Retro-futurism from a Mahogany
side-project; lightly-woven electronica gliding
towards a grand vision.

Five Songs by The Set Designers, by The Set
Designers (Penpal) – Swedish girl with an out-
of-tune guitar and heartfelt songs.

The Bobby McGees…Yes Please, by The Bobby
McGees (Cherryade) – Surreal and child-like
insights into the human condition, foul-
mouthed buffoonery and profound revelations.

Ordeal's Big Band, by DJ Ordeal (Sparticus
Stargazer) – Tape manipulation wizard scores
a perfect bullseye with reconstructed big band
sounds and telephone chimes.

A Hiding Smile, by Apple Orchard (Humblebee
Recordings) – Home-recorded loveliness recall-
ing (or imagining?) simpler and more innocent
times

Dreaming Out Loud, by Dear Nora (Magic
Marker) – Katy goes to her room with a bor-
rowed guitar and an 8-track. Twenty-four hours
later she comes back out with this beautifully
reflective collection.

Wintertime Queen, by The Butterflies of Love
(Fortuna POP!) – Deceptively loose stylishness,

carefully crafted sentiments. The B-side
"Complicated" is the real A-side here.

Christmas, by Blanket (Big Billy) – Deftly wielded
guitars and Vicky's beautiful voice. Simple,
lovely, and almost perfect.

Secret Home Party, by Various Artists (Little Pad)
– Compilation of American bands on a Tokyo
label. Ukele star Oliver Brown convenes a trio
that outshines the more established stars. In a
hand-made sleeve.

In The Devil's Garden, by The Castaway Stones
(Boa) – Jangling guitars and stylish vocals on
red vinyl with hand-drawn labels.

Italian Electro/Kumari, Split (Catmobile Singles
Club) – It's Kumari that make this special.
Clumsy wondrousness that made me want to
start my own label.

Aeba Suki Suki, by The Knockouts (Mademoiselle)
– Female beat combo with a '6os fascination,
the B-side is the hit on this one. The label was
run by a French girl living in London, releasing
records by Japanese girl bands with attitude.

When I Was Howard Hughes, by Hydroplane (Bad
Jazz) – A couple of strummed chords and a
drone, picked guitar reverb, and a yearning
voice – nothing else needed.

Chen Si

Every weekend, Mr Chen travels twelve and a half miles to the Yangtze River Bridge in Nanjing and walks, or rides his scooter, along its length. The bridge is said to be the world's most prolific suicide site, with over two thousand people having jumped to their deaths from it. The toll would be several hundred more if it wasn't for Mr Chen. He has been patrolling the bridge for many years. He looks out for possible jumpers and talks to them. Sometimes he physically prevents them from climbing over the bridge's barrier, but a few have slipped from his embrace to their deaths. He rents an apartment near the bridge where those who turn away from killing themselves can stay for a while. A volunteer team of psychology students from two local universities talk with them; Mr Chen says that stopping people from jumping is only the first step in helping them with their problems. He comes to the bridge on his days off – his wife complains about how much time he spends there, and he couldn't afford to enrol his daughter in an advanced class at school because he has put so much money into his voluntary activities. A documentary film was made about him and released in 2016 – *The Angel of Nanjing*.

Halotus and Sporus

Halotus was a eunuch and the Chief Food-Taster to Emperor Claudius in Ancient Rome. There are suspicions that he was involved in a plot to murder Claudius. He is said to have been ordered by Agrippina, the Emperor's wife, to poison his food. After Claudius' death, Nero succeeded as Emperor.

Nero was a particularly debauched Emperor who took a strong liking to a pretty youth called Sporus. He had the boy castrated and married him, requiring his new wife to wear the full regalia of a Roman Empress. Once the Senate had declared Nero a public enemy and he had been killed, Sporus became the wife of the Prefect of the Praetorian Guard which had been involved in removing Nero. Sporus' new husband didn't last long, as he too was killed after plotting to assume the throne. Sporus then took up with a subsequent Emperor, Otho, whose short reign also ended with his violent death. The new Emperor, Vitellius, proposed to parade Sporus in public and have him raped and then killed as part of a gladiator show. Sporus took his own life rather than be humiliated in this way – it is thought that he was still only a teenager when he died.

The Kizlar Agha

This translates as Master of The Girls and was the most senior position that a eunuch could hold in the Ottoman court. It was also one of the highest offices in the imperial hierarchy. The post was created in 1574 and for over three centuries it was held exclusively by Africans, as only black eunuchs were permitted entry to the most restricted areas of the palace. They were responsible for the supervision and administration of the inner heart of the empire. Not only did this bestow close proximity to the Sultan, but also to the wives and mothers of the ruling family, who themselves often possessed a great deal of power. The most senior white eunuch held the less influential position of Kapi Agha (Master of The Gate) and did not have a similar level of access to the private centre of the imperial court. The Kizlar Agha held a great deal of political power at various points in history, and was also responsible for the charitable foundations which funded the upkeep of the holy cities of Mecca and Medina.

Cornered

You never know what's around the corner, especially if you avoid turning it. Come on, one foot in front of the other, you can do it. Let's see what's there.

Intimacy

Nowadays there is a term that is used to describe a certain kind of sexual behaviour preference – demisexual. It means someone who cannot become aroused without feeling an intimate connection with a partner. I'm pleased that there is now a name for how I was; it makes it seem valid. I used to think that I was just repressed, or that there was something wrong with me, because I didn't wish to have casual sex with strangers like normal people were supposed to do. My later use of pornography, after my castration, only increased a sense of alienation within me as its portrayal of sexual activity is disconnected and purely mechanical in nature, and usually bereft of genuine human feeling. These days I often fantasise about being with a woman and *not* having sex with her – we cuddle and caress, sharing an emotional intimacy. When I first used a 'phone sex service I would exchange descriptions and evocations of real sex with the girl operative; neck-kissing, hair-stroking, gentle murmurs of arousal. I never "got off" by doing this, but it might illustrate that my truest and deepest desire was for closeness, rather than climax achievement.

Sei Shonagon

She was a lady of the Japanese imperial court over a thousand years ago. I very much enjoyed her *Pillow Book*, a loose collection of observations, gossip, and reflections. Ms Shonagon wrote her pieces over several years, during a period when Japan was beginning to move away from the influence of China. The official language used in documents at the time was a hybrid of Chinese and Japanese, which women weren't permitted to learn. They were restricted to Japanese, which was seen as being a "common" language then. Consequently, a lot of the earliest Japanese literature is written by female authors.

In *The Pillow Book*, there is mention of morning after letters. Apparently, gentlemen and ladies of the court were banned from consorting with each other, but there were also rules governing this forbidden, but regularly occurring, behaviour. The gentleman was expected to visit the lady in her chamber and had to leave before sunrise. He was also required to write a note that morning and have it delivered to her with a spray of cherry blossom or other flowers. The message was expected to take the form of a poem written upon fine paper in praise of the recipient's feminine wonderfulness. I read a suggestion somewhere that some ladies may have dismissed lovers because they did not consider their poetry to be of an acceptable standard.

After I'd read *The Pillow Book*, I began thinking that

perhaps even someone like me might be able to produce a "book" of some sort.

Ottoman Eunuchs

In the fifteenth century, the Ottomans took control of Constantinople and Byzantium. Eunuchs continued to serve many functions in the new empire. The Koran forbade castration, but eunuchs were brought from Christian sources. White eunuchs were imported from the Balkans or the Caucasus whilst, black eunuchs were transported from Abyssinia, now known as Ethiopia. Only black eunuchs were permitted to enter the harem; most of these came from a single Coptic monastery, Abou Gerbe, in what is now Egypt. Boys were captured from Abyssinia and Sudan and taken to the monastery, where they were chained to a table and had their sexual organs removed with a knife. They were then buried up to their necks in hot sand with a piece of bamboo inserted into their urethra. The mortality rate was reported to be very high; those that survived were greatly prized and fetched high prices at slave markets.

Lover Boy

As a young man, I was little more than a series of conditioned gestures. I was psychologically neutered and acted in accordance with an idea of how I was *supposed* to behave. I was in love with an idea of romantic love and believed that sex was a beautiful and special thing that you shared with someone you cared about very much. I wished to be a considerate and caring lover – when I was with a girl you could almost hear the orchestra playing in the background as I performed in another big production. I actually *did* enjoy being gentle, sweet, and affectionate though. When I had balls, I didn't really know what I wanted for myself sexually but was aroused by my partner's arousal. I enjoyed intimacy, but I think lots of women prefer a guy to be a real man in the bedroom; a bit of a beast who takes what he wants. I was too repressed to be like that, too tame and timid. Whilst I strove to be an attentive and responsive lover, I could never give women the deep shiver of raw excitement that they enjoy experiencing.

Realisation

I am a shadow that wishes to be annihilated by the light, a hologram that craves substance – a corpse in search of life.

Self-Abuse

It seemed okay to bully myself; it's not as if I was hurting anyone that mattered. I had to take out my anger on someone. I relentlessly beat myself every day, and no-one ever had any idea of the damage I inflicted upon my victim. Though I was nobody, I still had power over somebody – even if it was only me.

Chaste Lechery

Some people say that the brain is the most powerful sexual organ of all, and that sex is really "all in the mind". I might look at a woman and the switches in my head click, but nothing happens. If I try to fantasise about her, abstract images may be conjured in my imagination, but still nothing happens – the mental circuits that initiate desire have no effect. These triggers can sometimes create ghosts within non-existent machinery which haunt me. Attraction itself becomes a pleasurable objective, one which arouses a phantom desire within me. This occasionally becomes a repetitive loop in my brain, feeding back onto itself, creating a magnetic field of unreleasable charge which torments me.

Cheap Love

Love has no intrinsic value, it's worth is set by market variables – like everything else in our culture, it is a commodity. A small amount of love from a high-value individual is more desirable than a lot of love from a low-status person. There is a glut of unwanted love in our world, and it becomes toxic and poisons the hearts of those that carry it inside them.

Self-Medication

Oh, woe is me. I'm such a hidden treasure, so unjustly neglected. I'd be a real catch for some lucky lady, but nobody wants me – which just shows how unfair the whole world is. There! A little pity pill always makes things better, doesn't it?

Random Insignificances

Near The Blue Pig, a man pastes a large advertising poster on a billboard. We ask him if his is the sort of job where training is given, or you learn as you go along. We also wonder if it's like putting up wallpaper. He seems pleased to chat for a while and explains that the paste is thinner than for wallpaper and the paper of the posters is wet. He'd learnt "on the job" and has been doing this for twenty years. You note that he seems to be rather accomplished, but he replies that he just isn't any good at anything else. We don't believe him.

Somehow, we find ourselves in a shiny store – how did we get here? This is a dead-zone of miserable consumption, a strip-lighted battery farm for consumer grazing. People wander, blank-faced and dead-eyed, between racks and shelves, looking for something unnecessary and pointless to buy. We see ourselves in an unexpected mirror – we look just the same as everyone else. Quick, let's get out. We won't find what we're looking for here.

Piccadilly Gardens – a girl communicates in sign language whilst speaking Spanish to a young chap. A homeless guy studies a music score in his lap; the next time we pass he's playing a tin whistle.

A middle-aged couple walk along Oxford Road; he says something and smiles. She stops suddenly, grabbing his arm. She stretches up to him, he lowers his head. They kiss quickly, and then continue walking. She smiles happily and looks straight ahead. I try not to be jealous of him…and fail.

A girl with the *coolest* gold trainers walks along Oldham Street as if it's a scruffy catwalk. Lo-fi style, high-spec attitude – top marks.

A man sits outside Cafe Cotton playing a saxophone. He's a cabdriver; the car sits empty and quiet by the kerb.

The tune sounds vaguely familiar, suggesting rich invisible harmonies. When he pauses for a moment, you ask him what he was playing. "I don't know, just something that came to me" – I tell him that it sounds good. His name is Keith – he'd stopped for a coffee and felt the urge to blow a little. I'm glad he did.

Two Chinese girls wait at the crossing on Princess Street. There is no traffic at all, but they won't step onto the road until the green man says it's okay. What's the hurry anyhow?

A girl races across Salford Crescent in the dark, running fast. She sprints towards the bus stop with her arm extended. The driver sees her but closes the door and pulls away; she holds out her hands in forlorn appeal. Chalk up another hollow victory to petty unkindness.

A disassembled guitar has been placed carefully against a fence near Halle St Peters. Disjointed and separate pieces construct an abstract whole. We keep looking at it to make sure that it is really broken; it still seems alive, capable of making beautiful music.

A man stands stiffly in St. Peter's Square; he has a hearing aid in his left ear. He carries a small bag that has "Perfume as Art" on it – a present for a lady. He's really nervous, she's making him wait. We hope that the evening will go well for them.

The canal is leaking from the bridge across Store Street; a stream runs down the bank, across the pavement, and into a drain. The pavement is covered in a green slime and it's slippery to walk upon. Just like under the Station Approach Bridge.

In All Saints Park, there is a long tape suspended between two trees, about three feet from the ground. I wonder if it is an art installation, some sort of security or crowd control equipment. Soon a young man steps onto it and walks its length; ah, a slackline. He seems quite at home there and has very good balance. Soon some girls come and watch him, he smiles at them. Then more girls approach and one asks if she can have a go. He holds her hand, with discreet chivalry, giving support as she wobbles and makes uncertain progress. Her friends film the scene on their 'phones. A few hours later in St Peter's Square we recognise the young dash once more, his line is suspended between two trees. He elegantly traverses it whilst holding an umbrella, thick long curls dance under his hat. Soon girls are stopping to watch him once more – he seems to be quite an attraction for young ladies.

Spring has sprung. We sit in Parsonage Gardens, one island in a small archipelago of urban green. A magnolia has begun to bloom. We stroll to the Irwell and lean against the rail, looking at the triangular building on the other bank. Up high a man and woman sit on a balcony smoking cigarettes and chatting. Along from us, three tents are pitched on a dead-end walkway. A distracted chap comes, calling out names. He quickly unzips the entrance to each tent but they're empty, he leaves to continue his search elsewhere.

There is so much construction going on at the moment. Play the crane game; stand on one spot, then a three-hundred-and-sixty-degree turn and sweep, how many can you count? I've got into the twenties a few times.

In May, greenish-yellow goslings walk uncertainly across the towpath, or swim awkwardly upon the canals, tweeting excitedly. Protective parents keep a close eye upon them as well as passers-by.

We sit on the steps of the back entrance to the Town Hall; a couple of homeless guys come and sit beside us when it starts to rain. They smoke roll-ups and discuss the existence of God, amongst other things. We go to the newsagent and buy some tobacco for them; they wish us a good day.

One summer someone attached large pieces of cardboard to the railings on Salford Crescent. On these were painted letters that spelt a message – You Are Beautiful!

Bus drivers seem to enjoy accelerating along the stretch of Oldham Street between Forbidden Planet and Cow, even when the lights are red, and they'll have to brake very sharply to stop in time. Perhaps it gives them pleasure to see pedestrians scamper out of their way, one day someone won't be quick enough, and the driver will have scored a hit.

A young man asks us for directions. He can barely speak any English; I think he's trying to get to Piccadilly Station perhaps. He talks on his mobile to someone in Arabic and gives me the 'phone, a voice asks me to direct him to the bus station. It's not far, so I say to come with us, he follows. We talk to him whilst we walk but he doesn't understand anything we say. We turn a corner and there it is, he says – "Thank you" and shakes our hands. Let's hope he knows where he's trying to get to.

Raindrops upon the canal, and puddles as well. A mesmeric pattern that is always beautiful to behold, a rippling of consciousness. Watch for a while, time becomes stationary; you become part of the stillness too. If you look and see it in the right way, that is.

We watch people's faces as they pass in the street. They wear bland masks, but their features come alive when they talk to someone or miss the light at the crossing. Sometimes we catch the eye of a fellow observer, someone else who watches people.

At the place where the narrow canyons of Thorniley Brow and Well Street converge, a group congregate and wait patiently, some with tents and bags. Eventually the dealer arrives and stands on the corner step whilst his mate keeps a watch. The buyers cluster around him, coins and notes are quickly exchanged for little plastic bags, then they disperse with urgent intent. Cooking up is conducted between nearby cars, trousers are dropped, injections completed quickly. The used syringes lie scattered amongst the litter, the faeces, and the broken glass.

In St. John's Square an old lady feeds the pigeons; they gather at her feet, on the bench which she's sitting on, over her thighs and onto her lap. It looks like she has a moving grey blanket draped over her legs to keep her warm.

A boy fishes for pike in the canal near the new Urban Splash development in Ancoats; he's caught three before, he tells us. His mother is fishing too, about twenty yards around the corner where the boats are moored. We watch a shoal of tiddlers glide beneath the surface – later we see a lot of fry sheltering in very shallow water. The houses were prefabricated and shipped in, but the apartments are being built onsite at a tremendous rate. The construction workers finish their shift, the crane driver climbs down from his cab, the hook hanging from the crane continues to swing gently once everyone has gone. The site falls quiet, a black and white cat tiptoes slowly along the bank. The sky becomes darker and the breeze picks up – there's rain coming. It's needed, it's been too hot and sunny for the last few days.

Shining pavements, silver rooftops, a dark sky. Umbrellas with legs, leaning into the rain. On the bus upstairs windows become opaque, water drips from your coat, close your eyes…and open them. Sunshine, it's hot inside the Anthony Burgess window, like a greenhouse. A girl rides pillion on a bicycle as her boyfriend pedals standing up along Cambridge Street. Shall we have another piece of lemon drizzle?

A young thin guy walks along Cheetham Hill Road. He's wearing black and has an old guitar; it's strapped around his neck and shoulder as though he's about to step onto a stage to play. There are no amplifiers on the pavement though. He looks so happy, anticipating the moment when he will plug a lead into his newly acquired instrument. He'll tune it perhaps, and then…oh yes!

A little girl has fallen, she cries whilst her mother crouches in front of her and pulls a tissue from her coat pocket, speaking soothingly. Bags with shopping spilling out from them lie abandoned on the ground, temporarily forgotten. The sobs subside, Mummy can fix anything.

On Oldham Road at the car wash a man performs balletic movements as he power-sprays a big black four-wheel drive. Two sullen guys vigorously wipe the bodywork of a second car with sponges, whilst a couple of disinterested girls dry a third with chamois. There's a crumbling building nearby, beside a big tree with a large nest sitting in the high branches.

The River Medlock flows behind the Lass O'Gowrie and beneath Oxford Road. During a late summer evening we watch bats fly back and forth over the river's course; a bird skims over the surface – a wagtail you think.

A girl crosses Hilton Street and is almost hit by a private hire minibus which is turning from Newton Street. The driver had been frustrated by having to wait whilst oncoming traffic passed, and the lights had changed by the time he accelerated. He jammed on his brakes just in time. The girl is restrained, only slightly raising her voice whilst she suggests that it might be a good idea if he watches where he's going in future. The chastened driver apologises, and then she strolls off as if nothing has happened – a rather cool young lady.

We sit outside the CHIPS building for a while; the breeze is very pleasant. The clouds shift eternally, each momentary pattern infinitely unique. The shouts of children blend with the quacks of ducks. A young couple walk past slowly, holding hands, murmuring softly to each other.

In Albert Square, one spout in the Thirlmere Fountain is set incorrectly; water sprays beyond the lip of the fountain onto the pavement. A boy, about twelve, and his father kick a ball back and forward between each other over the cobbles. A horn blares, a black shiny car at the lights; a Deliveroo cyclist engages in angry conversation with the driver. The driver gets out, stands face-to-face, gets back in his car and drives off. A few people congregate around the cyclist, shaking heads and pointing here and there. It seems that the driver was a complete prick – there are quite a few of them in Manchester. A man and woman stroll by, her shoes are too big, they slip off her heel with each step, but she doesn't appear particularly concerned by this.

We hear someone shouting near a bus stop on Anson Road; a bus pulls away then slows to a halt. The doors open and three young guys sprint to get aboard, gasping heavily. So, there are some kind bus drivers after all. I'm pleased by this discovery.

Tramspotters collect numbers neatly in small notebooks at Piccadilly Gardens and Shudehill as carriages trundle past. They dislike being approached by outsiders enquiring about their secret endeavour. They see messages that the rest of us don't.

The hum of traffic, fragments of mobile telephone conversations, the toot of trams – the music of the city.

Today, it somehow makes perfect sense.

The Angel's Share

Once a whisky has been distilled, it is placed in wooden barrels and left to mature. Years later, when the barrels are opened for the final product to be bottled, they contain a much smaller volume. This is due to evaporation of the alcohol; the old distillers used to say that the vaporised whisky had risen to heaven where it was enjoyed by the angels.

A beautiful woman can be intoxicating, more powerfully so than any mere alcohol. I may never again sip from a glass, but sometimes if I breathe the air as she passes, I may still get a little tipsy.

A True Story

1. Boy meets girl.
2. Boy falls in love with girl.
3. Girl falls in love with boy.
4. They live happily ever after.

It *is* a true story, because it's happened a few times, here and there. It's a bit like the lottery though; you know that you'll never win it, but someone does.

Impostor

I go to music gigs, literature, or other artistic events and enjoy feeling that I'm a part of these occasions. I'm stimulated by the creative energy of others, delight in the radiance that is emitted by those more gifted than me. Sometimes I forget who I am for a little while, become lost in the magic, but soon realise once more that I am just a shabby gate crasher to the party, a talentless misfit who doesn't really belong amongst such company.

Conjecture

We all understand that time can seem to "stand still" or "race by"; perhaps it doesn't exist in a constant state. Time might be considered a variable constituent of the physical aspect of the universe. It may expand continuously in one direction at varying rates until it effectively contracts back upon itself in another plane. Eventually different factors coincide, and everything will be compressed into one point where all time and matter occurs simultaneously. This will initiate a "big bang", which is a cyclical event, not a single occurrence. Maybe time is an illusion that we use to chart existence and to navigate the universe.

Wonderful Things

A seventh chord played on an old guitar…a washing line with white sheets flapping on it during a breezy summer day…flowers growing in cracks of the pavement…waking up with someone lovely beside you…thick, soft woollen socks…a piece of chocolate melting in your mouth…when your laughter condenses into wispy clouds on a winter's day…a surprise meeting with an old friend…a teaspoon being carefully rested upon a saucer after the cup's contents have been stirred…

A Small Thing

I have much to be grateful for, and I try to appreciate my blessings. Yet no matter how I attempt to look at the big picture, my attention returns to the small thing that has been the cause of so much unhappiness for me. The sexual aspect to our being may only be a minor part of who we are, but it is an integral one. After my castration, I attempted to quarantine the damaged part of my psyche, to isolate it so that it would not infect the rest of me. This was the worst response to the situation I could have chosen; it only increased the destruction that resulted. The toxic material grew stronger, then leaked out and poisoned the parts of me that I had attempted to protect with my misguided solution. I fear that I am beyond repair now.

Walking in the City

I've always enjoyed going for long walks in cities. I did so long before I heard about Psychogeography. I just liked moving within the urban kaleidoscope, watching people and feeling part of the city – it has a soul, with many moods. I'm no psychogeographer, just a romantic wanderer who discovers something elusive by becoming lost in the city. I have no interest in conceptual walking; such as allowing algorithms to guide the route or using maps for different cities to negotiate the one you're strolling around. This betrays a rather self-regarding cleverness and is disrespectful. You insult the city by treating it in such a manner – it will shrug off your violations with indifference, but your foolishness will cost you. The city has much to reveal to you, but it will not do so if you are smug; a little humility is required. You must realise and accept your own insignificance; you are a tiny part of a multitude, moving through streets and buildings. Once you have lost an illusory sense of self you may connect with the vibrant energy that flows along the unseen neural pathways of the city. We like to believe that we go where we wish, but it is actually the city that suggests our footsteps – we follow as we are gently directed. That is why if the city trusts you, it will reveal more of itself and indicate new ways to hidden wisdoms.

Aimlessness is the purpose; there is no plan, no expectations. You find the way by becoming lost.

Sea Birds

A solitary black-browed albatross with a seven-foot wingspan was first spotted off the Scottish coast in the late 1960s. It is thought that the bird may have been caught in a storm and blown over the equator – the species is normally only found in the southern Atlantic. The individual was christened Albert and was seen many times over the next four decades vainly looking for a mate; but he was searching in the wrong hemisphere. On several occasions, he was observed attempting to woo much smaller female gannets who invariably spurned his advances.

Conservationists placed concrete replica gannets on an uninhabited island off New Zealand and played recordings of the bird's call to encourage real gannets to settle there and start a colony. One took up residence and was christened Nigel; he lived on his own there for several years. He unsuccessfully courted one of the artificial birds, built a nest for her, groomed her unyielding coat, and chattered forlornly to the unresponsive object of his affection. Eventually more gannets came to the island too, but Nigel didn't bond with them and died shortly after their arrival.

A male, called Rob by local conservationists, unsuccessfully sought a mate each year for a decade in a royal albatross colony near Otago, raising speculation about why he was seemingly so unattractive. Recently though it was noted that he had finally paired up with a female. Maybe happy endings do happen occasionally?

Refractions

The streets begin dancing, imperceptibly at first, but their movements increase gradually. Buildings shift, move, and change shape. The old patterns become distorted into startling new ones, which soon change again into something else. Colours merge until there are no colours anymore, just light – brighter, more intense. Our bodies fall away and are forgotten, along with the flimsy myths of their lives. We clung to them determinedly, too attached to foolishness for our own good. I am you; you are me – we are all each other. The old us would have scoffed, but we knew deep in our hearts all along that it was there all the time whilst we ignored it. We are going home, and now we disappear into the light – the beautiful, blissful light.

Nyguen An

Eunuchs were prevalent in Vietnamese and Korean empires of the past. Nyguen An was Vietnamese and sent as tribute to the Chinese Emperor in the fifteenth century. A skilled architect, he was instrumental in the construction of the Forbidden City. He was a hydraulics specialist who oversaw several innovative projects and the rebuilding of Beijing's fortifications.

Very Witty Eunuch Quotes

Critics are like eunuchs in a harem; they know how it's done, they've seen it done every day, but they're unable to do it themselves. – Brendan Behan

Being a writer in a library is rather like being a eunuch in a harem. – John Braine

A eunuch is a man who has had his work cut out for him. – Robert Burns

Urban Mood

Why do people take delight in being horrible to each other? Everyone seems very angry about being alive, and is keen to spread the misery around. Petty contempt is the default setting for interpersonal exchanges. Being unpleasant to someone else doesn't really make anything better, does it? I shall continue being a gentle renegade and display courtesy and consideration to my fellow humans today, so there! Take *that* rudeness – you will not win.

Byzantine Eunuchs

Emperor Constantine moved the imperial capital to Byzantium after the fall of Rome. The eastern remnant of the Roman Empire became a successful power in its own right for a thousand years until it fell to the Ottomans in the fifteenth century. There was extensive use of eunuchs in the imperial court, rich households, in the army and in the clergy. In the imperial court they fulfilled administrative, advisory and security roles. Many served as soldiers and were considered to be equally brave in battle as normal men. Originally the church frowned upon castration, but the eastern orthodox faith later permitted eunuchs to become monks and join the clergy. On a few occasions individual eunuchs effectively held supreme power briefly within the empire, but all came to a brutal end in the manoeuvrings that were a regular feature of imperial politics in Constantinople.

The Sweet Taste of Sadness

Quite often in the past, I would buy a large tub of ice-cream, sit down at the kitchen table and eat it all in one go. The melancholy realisation would then come to me that I had just experienced the highlight of the day.

Enthusiasm

I greatly prize enthusiasm in other people. I am very taken with someone who has a genuine and unaffected love for their interest or passion. You see their face light up when they talk about the pursuit or endeavour that absorbs them and fills them with happiness. Even if you know little of the subject, it's still quite inspiring to listen to them explain and discuss the cause of their enthusiasm. To do so is to hear an expression of love and to connect with an energy of aliveness that we all have within us. Sometimes this life force comes out in quirky and odd ways and should be appreciated all the more for this.

Once enthusiasm goes over into obsession or compulsion it quickly loses its charm; it will then become something narrow and small. Some passions have a dark, destructive side but childlike enthusiasm is a positive manifestation of our common being that enriches the world. I'm very attracted to those that become lost in their enthusiasms and discard constricting cynicism, opening out into a small beautiful bloom of humanity. I like those who love books, art, music and sport particularly, but also greatly enjoy the company of others with more obscure devotions.

In many cases, enthusiasm has greater value than ability. Some people who are technically adept at playing, performing, or creating don't seem to derive much pleasure from their talent. It can be quite touching to see the joy that those with less ability exhibit when they are doing what they love, however clumsily or ineptly. Their limitations only enhance the beauty of their endeavour.

Eric Newton

Eric was a jazz musician who worked as a postman and park gardener. He used to take a lot of tranquilisers, but eventually found more peace in running; he took part in many marathons whilst playing a saxophone to raise money for charities. In the 1970s he was depressed, possibly suicidal, and had no-one to talk to. He dialled numbers on the telephone at random and ended up speaking to someone in Melbourne. He asked the person what it was like there and they replied that the sun was shining bright and it was hot. Eric explained that where he was it was cold and dark; they chatted for a while. Eric asked if he could call again and the kind-hearted person at the other end said yes. They shared many further conversations and Eric eventually went to visit one day years later.

Zhao Gao

The Qin dynasty was a short-lived one that existed over 2,200 years ago, but the first to rule over a unified China. The Qin defeated the Zhao kingdom, one of the seven warring states, and Zhao Gao was castrated as a boy by the victors. He later served in the Imperial Palace and worked his way up the ranks and held a position of great power when the Emperor died. He was involved in a conspiracy with Premier Li Si to falsify the late Emperor's will and change the accession. This caused Crown Prince Fusu to commit suicide, and his younger brother Huhai ascended the throne, as the conspirators desired. Zhao Gao later treacherously ordered the execution of Li Si and his family. Then, he arranged for the assassination of Emperor Huhai, so that Fusu's son, Ziying, would be installed upon the throne. Ziying knew how wicked Zhao Gao was and had him killed before he could plot his downfall too.

Daggers in My Heart

Sometimes it's too much; the slightest gesture tears through my flesh and inflicts a sickening pain. A man puts his arm around his wife absentmindedly whilst they talk to a friend that they've unexpectedly bumped into. A girl leans against her boyfriend and rests her head upon his shoulder whilst listening to a band at a gig. A couple walk along the street holding hands, another couple kiss each other goodbye.

A cold, hard blade thrusts deep into me, is twisted – the bitterness rises up again.

The Loveliest Girl in Manchester

If she knew, I think she would probably be quite disgusted – so it's a good thing that she's never going to know. She works somewhere that I regularly pop into. Even if she wasn't employed there, I'd frequent those premises anyway, but it always makes a visit better if she's around. She's bookish, wears glasses, and is very smart and articulate. Sometimes she stands with her legs crossed, in the way that some young woman do, without realising how appealing they are being. She occasionally dresses like a frumpy schoolteacher, actually, but manages to carry it off with a natural style that makes her really rather cool. She genuinely doesn't appear to have the slightest idea how awesome she is. She's over twenty years younger than me and I have a secret crush on her. You want to vomit now, don't you?

Afternoon Delight

I like going to concerts and gigs that are held during the day; the effect of the music lasts longer than it does at evening performances. Usually you just go home and get into bed soon after experiencing music at night, and the next morning it has gone, but afternoon music will continue affecting you throughout the day, even if you don't realise it.

The Unwritten Book

The most wonderful of all literary creations, it contains the distilled sum of everything; all knowledge, experience and wisdom. It's widely available, in many versions. This leads to a certain amount of dispute and confusion – which is the *definitive* version? Actually, it doesn't matter at all, but people still argue endlessly about this question. Readers seem to experience vastly variable responses to the book. It's far too big to ever be completely read by any single individual, but many of the chapters are individual books in themselves. The order of chapters, paragraphs and even sentences and words appears to be fluid and constantly changing. This can lead to confusion but is also, perhaps, the most sensible arrangement for such a work. Sadly, many are ignorant of its beauty and power, its very existence in fact. This most wonderful creation has no known author, although many theories have been advanced concerning possible identities. The writing is unutterably beautiful, deceptively light and simple, yet profound and deeply moving. It requires no translation; it can be understood by anyone. The work may occasionally be encountered in greatly abridged and truncated editions, and mis-leading claims are often made of these being the entire book itself in codex form – impossible! They are just brief abbreviations which can lead to a distorted per-ception and understanding, and can be widely variable depending upon the selected material. It is best when encountered in the most fragmented loose-page form, as though it was thrown up in the air to be scattered by the wind over land and time. The most unusual feature of this great work is that it has no explicit text. Each page is formless and blank, or appears so, yet perusal at cer-tain times leads to intense responses being experienced within astute and receptive readers.

Narcotic

Anger is the drug of our times, a toxic stimulant that is powerfully addictive but causes great harm. It provides an illusion of clarity, moral righteousness, and self-value to those who are under its spell. Users feel greatly pumped up whilst it combusts within them, but it is a poison that destroys from inside, as well as the cause of great damage when it dictates people's actions. Instead of empowering those under its influence, it enslaves them and keeps them in an emotional servitude that is increasingly difficult to escape from. Once there was said to be an opiate of the masses that kept them docile, now there is an over-supply of a more dangerous drug that keeps the general population under the yoke of continuous rage.

Fair Exchange?

The average life expectancy for men in this country is just under eighty years old. It might be that I could reasonably hope to have over twenty years to live. If I could, I would gladly swap those for just two years of being young, healthy, and virile.

A Hidden Suffering

I tried to avoid having uncomfortable thoughts about women, sex, and love but they only became more powerful because of my attempts to subdue them.

Usually I noticed women in a disconnected way, but every now and then my psychological hard drive would become full with all the feelings that I had repressed, and it would take no more. A random woman would be the catalyst for the release of all the suppressed emotions and the hard drive was violently wiped clean once more. I knew that sweet thoughts would bring disaster, but it was too late as I'd begun to fantasise about her. This caused a blow-back of toxic emotions – self-hatred, despair, shame and anger. I attempted distraction strategies; shovelled food into myself to the point of discomfort, went for long walks, desperately tried to immerse myself in music, art, or pornography. Nothing ever worked, so I just rode out the storm as best I could. At such times I thought about jumping from high rooftops to put an end to my suffering. I became nihilistic and resentful; I knew that this was wrong and felt guilt for my self-indulgence, causing me to heap more condemnation upon myself and further increase my agony. Eventually the storm subsided, and I would step out from my flimsy shelter to view the battered and desolate landscape that remained.

The Grass Isn't Always Greener

One evening at the Wonder Inn, I got into a conversation with an amusing chap who was a bit tipsy from a few drinks. He suddenly confided that he was lonely and then he opened up to me, so I listened. He told me that he'd built up a successful business and then sold it, he and his wife had divorced, and his children had grown up and left home. Nowadays, he went out in the evenings and wandered around bars in town on his own. He said that he had no problems getting ladies but, whilst a guy might need a shag every now and then, none of the women he picked up were looking for a deeper relationship. He suggested that women were mainly interested in his money and didn't really want love. I replied that there were probably more than a few good women out there who would be very happy to share a loving relationship with him, and that he would find one of them someday. I later chuckled at the idea of me giving anyone advice about such matters, but it also occurred to me that if someone like him couldn't find love, what chance did I have? I saw him one last time that evening, as I left to go home; he was sitting at a table with two women who laughed with delight as he charmed them with his witty humour.

Whilst I was attending sessions with a sex-therapist, she referred to other clients occasionally to illustrate points that she was making. It became apparent to me that there was a man who was also seeing her who was wealthy and having lots of sex with many women – and he was miserable. I wondered which of the two of us led the unhappier existence.

Resentment

Often, when I see a happy couple together, it makes me smile. Sometimes, unfortunately, it can also make me feel resentful that I don't have what they do, that I have no-one to love. Resentment can be triggered when I hear people talk about sex, relationships, and love. I become more aware that I am unloved and unlovable. Being a witness to other people's small moments of joy can cause a sourness to rise inside me, observing other people's happiness is to have my nose rubbed roughly in my own misery. Sometimes just a small gesture, such as a girl reaching to hold her boyfriend's hand, can cause me pain.

Resentment is a destructive emotion, a constant picking at a scab that only prevents it from healing. It is to live in an imaginary place that offers the illusion of value based on a perception of injustice, but in fact it only degrades the sufferer. Often people resent another individual for particular reasons. A grudge is borne, nursed and nurtured against that person. My resentment is more general and impersonal, but just as destructive, perhaps more so for its vagueness. I resent guys who can have sex with their girlfriends, resent that they have girlfriends, resent that they have balls and I don't. I resent that they're men and I'm not. I resent that women keep falling for douchebags and arseholes. I resent those that have someone to love, who love them too, and who love each other.

I knew that resentment was bad and tried to pretend that I was above feeling it; perhaps this stopped me from dealing with it. I wouldn't admit that it rose up inside me, but now I have learnt a little, perhaps I can begin to do something about it.

Resentment can be an unacknowledged jealousy of those considered more fortunate, talented or beautiful than you. Life's not fair! We all know that, but at least you can get even with others by resenting them for their gifts, their opportunities, their happiness. Resentment is one member of a poisonous gang – some others are self-pity and anger. They have a close resemblance in their behaviour and effects, running wild and leaving destruction in the minds of those who allow this toxic team free rein to roam in their psyches. They destroy hope and optimism; by a refusal to forgive wrongs, imaginary or not, they create a false sense of power and value. The resentful will recite a list of grievances like a mantra so that they can remain in a state of reassuring unhappiness. Self-pity leads to resentment; resentment leads to anger. All of these lead to misery and pain.

Climbing

You climb the slope, just taking one step at a time – small steps, upwards. You breathe heavily, your legs ache, you stop for a moment. You turn around and look – how far you've come! The view is beautiful; you didn't realise it would look like this. You didn't believe you could climb this far, but you've come a long way by just taking small steps, one after the other. You have your breath back now, so you turn and take another little step, and then another…

Lost in the City

In town, people often look in bewilderment at their 'phone screens or at printed street maps of the city centre. I used to like asking them if they were lost and point them towards where they were looking for, often showing them the route to take on the pages of the A to Z guide of the city that I usually carried in my rucksack. I believed that I was being helpful to others in offering my assistance, but perhaps I was really only a sad busybody who didn't have a life and wanted to feel useful.

No More Mister Nice Guy

Sometimes a guy tries too hard with a woman and, though it might seem a strange thing to say, she deserves better than that. On the face of it, showing lots of consideration and affection might seem like a good thing, but sometimes it's not that simple. Perhaps he genuinely cares for her, but is also acting this way because he is subconsciously seeking affirmation from her. If so, it can then become more about him showing what a super guy he is than how special she is to him. He has confused the idea of being a good man with a series of virtuous gestures that are motivated by his emotional neediness and lack of self-value. He wants her to tell him that he's kind and considerate, that he's good and loving – he needs to be constantly reassured of his worth by her. He is acutely sensitive to criticism and will desperately avoid arguments. When rejection finally comes, as it usually does, it will hurt greatly because he genuinely doesn't understand what he's done "wrong". He may take refuge in self-pity and find a cold comfort in cynical clichés that suggest women don't want to be treated with respect by men.

I think I might know what I'm talking about in regard to this matter; I was a bit like this once – only I didn't realise it at the time. I would bring my girlfriends flowers, give them little presents and "surprises" that became so regular that they no longer surprised. I constantly gave compliments, was considerate and attentive – literally to a fault. Some "nice guys" are insecure and that's why they try too hard. They may be good-hearted and well-meaning, but their love is flawed and fragile, its quality weakened by meekness and self-doubt.

Unaddicted

I bought some books about porn addiction, and found one to be particularly useful. It contained questionnaires which could be used to assess levels of addiction; I completed these and was bemused to discover that I wasn't actually an addict. It wasn't until I attended counselling several years later that the therapist provided a correlating opinion by observing that I wasn't addicted to anything, but was isolated and lonely. I had confused regular use with addiction. When I used pornography, it was in a vain attempt to numb a pain that never went away.

Note to Self

You're a disgusting and revolting creep. How could you ever look a woman in the eye and tell her what you are? You'd only make her flesh crawl.

Unsent Letter

I wrote a letter to her – the woman that I would have loved if I'd remained a man. More honestly, I made several futile attempts to write this letter, producing various drafts that were discarded and destroyed. How could I say what cannot be said? You can imagine the clumsy clichés that were placed upon the paper with laughable reverence. I told her that I was sad that we hadn't met, but hoped that she had enjoyed a happy life, I told her how much I would have loved her if things had been different. I found out later that a similar exercise is a standard practice of grief counselling, but I can't say that it helped me in any noticeable way. So, it would seem possible that I was grieving for someone I never met and never knew. I sometimes wonder what she would have been like.

Don Ritchie

Don lived near The Gap, a coastal cliff overlooking Sydney Bay, and would often gaze out of his window at the beautiful view. This place was also one where many came to end their lives. He learnt to spot those that looked lost and without hope. He'd cross the road and stand beside them, smile and ask – "Is there anything I can do to help?" That was all it took to turn people around sometimes, away from suicide. He'd invite them back for a cup of tea or a beer at his house and chat with them, listening to their stories.

No-one knows how many people Don stopped from jumping. Official figures say one hundred and sixty, and other people suggest that it was a lot more. Late in life he was recognised with awards, but only said that he couldn't just watch people throw themselves off the cliffs and do nothing. He understood the power that a smile and a kind word possess, and the effect that these can have on people at the right time.

Grow a Pair

Man up and grow some balls? I wish it was that simple. Sometimes you hear people say – "fake it until you make it" – but pretending to be something doesn't make it real, no matter how hard you try. My secret shame burns like acid inside me.

Pretend

We all wear masks sometimes; it's easier to pretend everything's alright even when it's not. Sometimes we fool ourselves into thinking that we're not wearing a mask and that the artificial expression that we catch sight of in an unexpected mirror is our real true self. That's the dirtiest trick that you can play – you don't even realise that you're conning yourself. Pretending you're happy won't make you happy.

Young Love

I walk along Oxford Road. There are lots of people coming and going; a girl overtakes me. I notice that she has lovely, thick, dark hair and a superb figure before she disappears into the crowds. When I reach St. Peter's Square, I see her again, she's looking around for someone. Then, she walks quickly towards an approaching boy with a big smile upon her face. He's tall and athletic, lean and loose; he smiles as he bends forward to kiss her. They walk off holding hands; they both seem so *happy*. They look just right for each other, I think.

Self Destruct

I shunned the very thing that I wanted more than anything else. I felt that I was unworthy of being loved and closed my heart to the possibility of love ever coming into my life. I destroyed my own happiness and threw away future possibilities with a calamitous choice of attitude. I wish that I had not been so stupid and would like to have the chance to go back and start again. Life's not like that though, is it? You only get one tour around the carnival, and it is your responsibility to make the most of every moment and opportunity. I learnt too late; I hope you'll be wiser than I was.

Gang Bing

Regarded as the "patron saint" of Chinese eunuchs, he was a general who castrated himself to avoid accusations of impropriety with the imperial concubines. He was made chief eunuch by the third Ming emperor, and after his death was deified. He was buried on the outskirts of Beijing, and the surrounding plot of land was declared to be the final resting place for eunuchs and concubines. An ancestral hall was built there in his honour – it was later enlarged and became a Taoist temple. Over time, this became a place for retired eunuchs to see out their days. For the next five centuries, the site was known as The Eunuch's Temple, but after the communist takeover it was renamed The National Cemetery for Revolutionaries. High ranking officials and elite party members are now buried there.

Faking It

Sometimes I'd speak with a lady on the 'phone service and act out a scenario, having sham 'phone sex with her. I pretended to have an orgasm at the appropriate point in the charade. This is a *very* weird way to behave, don't you think? I was emotionally excited by having fake 'phone sex, as if acting out in this way allowed me to have a sense of sexual being that I could never have in reality. It was like having a fantasy about having a fantasy, which shows how wretched and pathetic I had become. In the scenarios I could pretend to be a virile man with balls. I'd ask her to play with these imaginary testicles as part of the performance – an impotent eunuch fantasising about being a man.

Fanzine

Home-made, DIY booklets and magazines – the name is a splicing of "fan" and "magazine", then often contracted to 'zine (pronounced "zeen"). These are unofficial amateur publications, often concerned with a specific subject which inspires enthusiastic devotion in, or has a deep personal interest for, the author, or authors. Typically, they have a cut and paste nature, with material appropriated from a wide range of sources which can be mixed with original text and pictures. Often, they are published in a photocopied format with variable production values. Some are quite beautiful; a good 'zine is truly a labour of love and may be the purest and most wonderful literary form of all.

An Ugly Rainbow

Mahatma Gandhi suggested that there were seven things that would destroy us –

    wealth without work
    pleasure without conscience
    knowledge without character
    religion without sacrifice
    politics without principle
    science without humanity
    business without ethics

Some of these seem to be in very plentiful supply at the moment.

Club di Giulietta

It's based in Verona – the setting for the Romeo and Juliet story. The heartbroken and the lovelorn have written to Juliet seeking advice for decades – each letter is read by a volunteer and replied to, if it is possible to do so.

Visitors to Juliet's house often leave letters and notes between the stones of its walls or write the name of loved ones on "Juliet's Wall". Some began writing their names, and those of their loved ones, on padlocks which were then secured to a gate at the back of the house. This began the custom of lover's padlocks being fastened onto the railings of bridges and gates that has spread across many European cities.

Eunuchs and Sex

Generally, it was considered that boys who were castrated before puberty did not feel sexual desire once they reached adulthood, as testosterone had not affected their development. Those castrated later in life, in adolescence and adulthood, retained impulses relating to sexual behaviour. Until the late twentieth century hormone replacement was not available but, despite this, some eunuchs who had a complete or partial penis could still experience erectile responses. Historically, most eunuchs were slaves, and therefore at the whim of their owners' wishes; sexual or otherwise. Most affairs and relationships were furtive and hidden – the capabilities of eunuchs were obviously restricted, but many still had a sexual aspect to their lives. Eunuchs were noted for the attentiveness and faithfulness that they displayed toward female partners. Most societies with eunuchs have left little record of their private lives, but documents relating to the imperial Chinese court suggest that eunuchs consorted with, and had full relationships with, a wide range of palace staff and courtiers, as well as, in some cases, members of the ruling family.

Some Places That I Heard Music

57 Thomas Street
Academy 3
The Art of Tea
Bakerie
Band on the Wall
Bangkok Bar
The Carlton Club
The Castle Hotel
Cord Bar
Creation Cafe (Angel Centre)
The Crescent
Crown & Kettle
Cuba Cafe
The Cutting Room
The Cornerhouse (Annexe)
The Deaf Institute
Dry Bar

Dulcimer

The Eagle Inn

The Egerton Arms

Fallow

First Chop Brewing Arm

Five Four Studios

The Flophouse (Bunker/White Hotel)

Fred's Ale House

Fuel

Gorilla

Guilty By Association

Gulliver's

Halle St. Peter's

Hot Bed Press

Hotspur House

International Anthony Burgess Institute

Islington Mill

The King's Arms

Klondyke Club

Kosmonaut

Kraak (Aatma)

Kro Bar

Le Classis

Lloyd's Hotel

Manchester Museum

Matt & Phred's

Mary & Archie's

The Music Box

New Bailey Arches
The New Oxford
Wolfson Reading Room (MCL)
Night & Day Cafe
Odd Bar
The Old Pint Pot
The Peer Hat
The Ritz
The Roadhouse
Royal Exchange Theatre
RNCM
The Ruby Lounge
St. Ann's Church
St. Chrysotom's Church
St. Phillip's Church
Salford Arms
Sandbar
Sound Control
The Spoon Inn
Strange Brew
SubRosa
The Soup Kitchen
The Star & Garter
Takk
Texture
The Thirsty Scholar
The Thompson's Arms
Three Minute Theatre

The Idea of It

Sometimes the idea of something that you have in your head is much better than the reality; the mythology is much more enchanting than the substance. You are enraptured by the fantasy. It shines brightly, but when you reach out to grasp it you already know that there will be nothing there. You always knew it, and it makes you sad. Yet you also understand that life is nothing without dreams, and that what you may become is perhaps dependent upon what it is that you dream about.

A Retard and a Fake

When I was a young man, I experienced retarded ejaculation in the earlier stages of a relationship; I was aroused and stiff but couldn't "finish" when having sex. This is a psychological problem, not a physical one. I was clearly repressed and was holding back on my own pleasure, trying too hard to please my girlfriends. I would get over this issue as the relationship developed and be able to come. Girls can take it very personally if you don't climax with them though, and you have to make it clear that she's very beautiful and ask her to be patient and understanding. I found that the problem persisted and became greater if my girlfriend made a big issue about it. I even ended up faking orgasms to avoid arguments, it's easy to do this when you're wearing a condom and the lights are off. This behaviour might demonstrate that I was already a psychological eunuch before I became one physically.

Say Hello, Wave Goodbye

A late autumn evening, it's cold and dark. A girl stops at the northern edge of Piccadilly Gardens; she has a case on wheels with an extended handle. She looks at the screen of her 'phone, whilst wearing her dead-eyed street face. She waits as the crowds pass by. A few minutes later a tall young man walks up behind her; he's well-dressed and handsome. He says something, she turns around and opens her arms wide and smiles with delight. He leans forward and kisses her, she hugs him elatedly. They walk off holding hands. She talks rapidly, the words tumbling from her mouth in a stream of happiness. He listens intently and smiles at her. They look great together; perfect in fact.

Later, I sit on one of the big benches in Saint Peter's Square. A young couple stroll together, holding hands, then turn and face each other. They kiss slowly before parting reluctantly. She walks towards the tram stop; he watches her go. Once she has climbed the ramp and reached the sheltered part of the platform, she turns around and smiles delightedly – he waited. They wave to each other, then he turns and disappears into the city. I am pleased that he didn't just head off immediately, as many young men would have.

Shadow

I cast a silhouette upon sunlit ground, yet have no substance. A vacuum of emptiness, distorting whatever light passes through me.

A Flag of Inconvenience

Eunuchs have a symbol which is seldom seen – a "broken arrow" variant of the Mars male symbol. It seems that there's also a eunuch's "pride" flag now too, although I can't really imagine anybody waving it with much enthusiasm. It is a tricolour; the central black panel has an orange eunuch symbol. The other two panels are different shades of yellow.

Clones

We like to think we're individuals; we're always trying to prove to ourselves how different we are from everyone else. All we really end up doing is confirming that we're all the same; whether we like to accept this or not. We are just clones acting in accordance with the programmes that are uploaded inside our heads. The software can easily be changed, is susceptible to corruption by viruses and other influences. Our individuality is a superficial illusion – we are just organic droids.

Kindness

It is the answer, it is always the answer. Sometimes it is the most difficult thing to find within yourself, but it is always there, and it is worth looking for.

When in Rome

Sometimes ancient Roman ladies shared their beds with eunuchs, the poet Martial wrote an intriguing couplet –
"Do you ask, Panychus, why your Caelia only consorts with eunuchs?
Caelia wants the flowers of marriage – not the fruits."

Comprehension

People talk about "the penny dropping", or an idea "dawning" upon someone – the moment when understanding arises in our consciousness. You try to understand something but can't "get your head around it". People try to explain the idea to you, but you don't "get it". Then, suddenly, you do. Where does that instant of comprehension come from and how does it arise? If you already had the capability to cause this shift within your mind, could it be that the code for understanding was already encrypted in your consciousness without you being aware of this? Even though you are absorbing external information, it makes no sense until electric circuits within your brain are arranged in a particularly appropriate manner.

Perhaps knowledge is often second-hand, acquired from external sources – facts and figures, words and images. Wisdom and understanding can only arise from within, and only if conditions are favourable for them to do so. Only you can bring about this moment of ignition, turn the handle that will open the door to an elsewhere. Sometimes, you must look so deeply within yourself that you go beyond yourself and achieve a brief glimpse of the universal consciousness.

Brief Interlude

1. Sit quietly for a moment
2. Close your eyes and breathe
3. Think of someone you love
4. Smile

Manchester Museum

It's part of the Manchester University building. I've been there for a poetry reading and a gig, and, in between listening to some unusual music there, once I got the chance to look at a fossilised lightning strike and some flexible sandstone. I was very impressed. Just along from the entrance to the museum is the Coupland Building, where Alan Turing did a lot of his work on computers and artificial intelligence. He underwent chemical castration in 1952 as a punishment for homosexual activity and died two years later, possibly by suicide.

The Emperor's Clothes

I get a bit bored with all the adulation that's heaped upon too many bands and performers from the past. Whilst some of them were good in their way, a lot of rubbish is spouted and written about their importance and influence upon civilisation. I really wish that a little boy would shout – "the emperor isn't wearing any clothes!" and everyone would realise what a lot of crap they've been worshipping for too long. I suppose some people need gods, and in a godless age, we continuously deify empty plastic figures, filling them with false meaning.

Note to Self

It's not much fun, being you, is it? It can't be when you're such a big fat loser with no redeeming features. It's a wonder that you ever bother getting out of bed, let alone leave the house.

Stand Up Comedy

I seem to be running out of options in the search for a cure for my impotence. I've been prescribed the usual drugs for erectile dysfunction, but they didn't really help me. These treatments, known as PDE-5s, are vasodilators that temporarily enhance the blood supply to the penis. Unfortunately, when I tried them, I discovered that I may indeed be a dickhead after all, as my face and neck became very flushed and hot, my nose was blocked, and I found difficulty in breathing. When I looked in the mirror, I saw a big crimson-faced tomato head looking back at me, and I can't honestly say that he was particularly handsome. I have also been prescribed a vacuum pump device and a cream, but these haven't made much difference either.

Testosterone

Widely regarded as being the "male" hormone, women also have it coursing around their bodies, though usually in much lower quantities than men. It is produced by the ovaries and adrenal glands, in a roughly fifty-fifty split, and has a direct effect upon female libido, amongst a few other things.

Men's testosterone levels are far higher on average. It is mainly produced by the testicles, about 95 per cent, and the rest is produced by the adrenal glands. It is classed into three categories; free testosterone, which is not bound to any proteins and is able to enter cells and interact with receptors, is biologically active, and has the greatest effect. Free testosterone constitutes 2 to 3 per cent of the normal total, the other two types are bound to different proteins and have less direct influence.

The effects of testosterone on physique, development, physiology, psychology and behaviour are widely reported. Research on this appears to almost exclusively concentrate upon its influence on males. It is believed to increase aggression and sex-drive, risk-taking and competitiveness, confidence and self-esteem. It is said to reduce depression and fatigue. Higher levels have been found to increase muscle mass and reduce fat, enhance erectile function and mental concentration. Whilst it is obvious to conclude that testosterone is an influential hormone, I also think that there's a fair bit of mythology being spun around it as well sometimes.

The End of the Ottomans

An Irish journalist, Francis McCullagh, was present in Constantinople at the time of the Young Turk Revolution, and later wrote a book about the fall of the Ottoman Empire in which he makes several mentions of eunuchs at the court. The chief eunuch, Djevher Agha, and the second most senior eunuch, Nadir Agha, were described as having been enemies for many years. Nadir proved helpful to the revolution's success, and was rewarded with a comfortable exile, whilst Djevher was brutally executed. The reporter noted that Djevher had shown a great affection for a beautiful slave girl and had lavished her with presents and attention. She was reported to have been heartbroken at the death of her admirer. McCullagh commented that eunuchs had a reputation for forming strong, if sometimes fanciful, attachments to women which could sometimes result in "strange friendships" occurring.

A Single Moment of Pure Being

In the third to last scene of *The Naked Civil Servant*, Quentin Crisp describes the happiest moment of his life – when some sailors surrounded him with good-natured admiration on the seafront at Portsmouth. It was the one brief instant when he was truly and completely himself and was accepted and appreciated for it.

There Are People Worse Off Than You

This is not really a helpful response when someone expresses pain or unhappiness. Using this phrase can be to slam a door in someone's face. Sometimes people say this to dismiss someone who has expressed personal suffering or pain because they do not wish to hear what they are saying; it's shutting them up and shutting them out. You might also say this to yourself as a way of avoiding facing up to uncomfortable feelings. Everyone knows that there are people with bigger problems than them, and whilst it is always good to retain some perspective and not become too self-absorbed, it is not wise to dismiss genuine problems because they're not the "biggest" ones that it is possible to have. If issues are swept under the carpet and ignored, they will only continue causing damage; it's better to fix them whilst it is still possible to do so. It might be too late otherwise.

Suggesting to someone that their problems are trivial and unimportant can be detrimental and harmful; it belittles them and their feelings. It might cause someone to feel that they lack worth because their pain is irrelevant or invalid. They may then become reluctant to talk about their feelings and bottle them up inside; this could lead to them becoming prey to shame, guilt, and self-loathing.

Eunuchs During the Ming Dynasty

It is estimated that the eunuch population in China may have numbered over a hundred thousand at various periods during the Ming dynasty. Although the imperial court issued stern warnings to discourage the practice, local landowners and gentry routinely castrated members of the lower social classes for various reasons. The imperial court preferred to be the sole agency for creating castrates and founded a battalion of these which, at its peak, consisted of almost ten thousand armed eunuchs. They were well-trained in various military crafts but were regarded with deep suspicion by generals and senior officials who considered them wilful and insubordinate. The Eunuch's Battalion displayed complete loyalty to the Emperor, though, which was a valuable asset to the imperial court during an era when there was constant plotting against whoever was currently on the throne. The Eunuch's Battalion contributed greatly to the stability of the Ming dynasty in otherwise turbulent times.

Message in a Bottle

One afternoon, I sat on an old bench surrounded with litter; nothing seemed to make much sense. I hurriedly scribbled on several sheets of paper, rolled the pages tight, and pushed them down the neck of a bottle. I screwed the top tightly shut and threw it into the canal. It began to rain heavily, I got soaked and went to shelter somewhere.

Somehow, much later, you found the bottle and discovered its secret message. Please tell me what it says; I never knew, even as I wrote it.

Unsung

I recall in the early 80s watching an American sit-com on TV one evening. This particular episode featured two characters in NYC. One was an uptown girl from a wealthy family and the other an odd little guy from downtown. The little guy was bald and overweight and had a quick humour – apart from that he was nothing special. He *really* loved the uptown girl though, loved her with all her faults. She had issues, and every now and then they'd get too much for her and she'd go on a bender and become a complete mess. When she got like that, she was a real nightmare; her friends and family wouldn't have anything to do with her, so she would go to the one person who was always there for her — the downtown guy. A pattern had developed; she would go to him when she most needed to be loved, she'd stay with him for a few days until she felt better, then she'd leave him…until the next time she had a meltdown. This time the little guy explained to her that he couldn't allow this cycle to continue, that he loved her, but if she was going to leave this time, he didn't want her to come back again. She listened to him, surprised by his resolve, then replied by singing a song. When she sang it, his determination disintegrated — they both knew that he just couldn't help loving her. I thought that it must be a very special song if it could do that to someone — even if just in a TV show.

I remembered the first line of the song and visited a middle-of-the-road record shop and began looking at the track-listings of many LPs until I found it on a *Vic Damone Greatest Hits* record. I bought it and listened to the song over and over again, learning the melody and words so that I could sing it gently to myself as I walked through the streets of the city. A few years later, I came across a 1920s songbook that contained a piano version of the song. I taught myself to read music, just good enough that I could work out some chords for guitar. That was over a quarter of a century ago. Maybe I guessed the wrong chords but I'm not going to change them now. I thought that one day I would sing the song to someone special, but I never did. I still play it sometimes, whilst sitting alone and dreaming.

Square

If you end up with a boring miserable life because you listened to your mum, your dad, your teacher, your priest, or some guy on television telling you how to do your shit, then you deserve it. – Frank Zappa

He's right. I was a conformist, law-abiding, little goodie-two-shoes, and I had an unhappy life as a consequence. I did what I thought was the right thing without actually knowing why the right thing was supposedly the right thing. At primary school the teacher would award gold stars for a good piece of work – a neat exercise jotter, a challenging task completed, a particularly noteworthy effort. I enjoyed receiving a shiny affirmation from authority figures; the smile and the pat on the back, the endorsement for being such a good boy. When I reached adulthood, I continued to seek metaphorical gold stars, and sought approval for being a virtuous individual. I didn't know who I was; I tried very hard to be who I thought I was supposed to be – an upstanding and good person. I strove to be someone who cared about and respected other people, acted selflessly in the interests of the greater common good, was a positive influence upon the world. I was conditioned to be an obedient droid, a fearful servant of an ever-critical God who was never satisfied with anything I did. I meant well, wanted to be the good guy in an imaginary movie of my life, but all I have ended up with is a dreary DVD of disparate fragments that make no sense; they capture only a smudgy sense of false hopes and lost opportunities. I followed the rules and gained no benefit by doing so, yet watched those who ignored and broke them enjoy rich and happy lives. All my little gold stars are just meaningless pieces of nonsense that won't save me from unhappiness.

Chen Ju

Castrated as a boy, he worked in the imperial library where he was responsible for acquiring new books. Later he gained great power as an imperial intelligence chief, in charge of spies and secret police, and proved to be a restraining influence upon the impetuous emperor. He was known for his rational mind and reasoning approach, deep respect for the truth, and devotion to duty. He was also noted for his unusually kind and humane character, as well as for a deep wisdom. He avoided the use of torture, which was a common tool of governance at that time and became extremely popular with the general population. He was one of the few eunuchs to have achieved a position of power who died from natural causes at a peaceful, old age.

Little Pieces of Marshmallow

One day the couple took a train to meet their granddaughter who had started university. After a little tour in the rain, they decided to pop into the Blue Daisy, and sat beside an old non-descript who read a book distractedly.

The young woman was just growing into an awkward confidence, keen to show off this wonderful new chapter in her life. She spoke breathlessly of new places, and new friends, and new experiences. The couple belonged to the old places that she had now outgrown. She told them stories, tripping over her words with enthusiasm. They listened to her, enchanted by the way she spoke now. Coffees were ordered. The old man had never seen mini-marshmallow bits on top before, a small detail of the big city that amazed him. Sophistication was thus formally bestowed upon the girl.

It was the quiet spaces between conversational paragraphs that were the most touching. The unsayable expressed in the silent language of love.

The small bird had beaten her wings, clumsily at first, and had flown to a magical place where she would make many discoveries. The old pair visited and were so proud of her; did she really have any idea how much they cared for her? I did, sitting beside them that afternoon. The couple had such aching tenderness for their child's little girl. Sometimes I remember and my heart cracks open.

Boston Corbett

The man who allegedly killed John Wilkes Booth – Abraham Lincoln's assassin. He was a hat maker by trade, and it is suggested that he may well have been "mad as a hatter" due to the Mercuric Nitrate that was used during the manufacturing process. He self-castrated to avoid sexual temptation once he stopped drinking alcohol and had become devoutly religious following the death of his wife during childbirth.

Xin Xiu Ming

One of the few eunuchs to have written a memoir; it has not been translated into English, unfortunately. He was also unusual in that he was married with children; he consented to be castrated at the age of nineteen so that he could enter service at the imperial court. He served there for over twenty years, and when China was declared a republic, he became the last abbot of the "Eunuch's Temple" in Beijing. He later negotiated favourable terms with the communists for the takeover of the establishment, and secured assurances regarding the treatment of those eunuchs under his care.

Denis Mukwege

Why would a gynaecologist win the Nobel Peace Prize? More people have lost their lives in the DR Congo than in any other conflict since World War Two; estimates vary up to over five million. Gang rape is used as a weapon of terror to humiliate and break family and social bonds – the sexual mutilation of women is routine. Dr Mukwege and his team at Panzi Hospital do their best to repair the victims. He has been outspoken in his criticism of all sides in the series of conflicts that have engulfed the country for over two decades. On one occasion, his family were taken hostage in their home as gunmen waited for him to return from work in the evening; they opened fire as his car arrived outside the house. The driver was armed and killed one of the assailants and injured another before being killed himself. Mr Mukwege survived but took his family out of the country for their protection. He later returned to ensure that his work at the hospital continued. One day, he turned up at his hospital in the morning to find some teenage girls waiting at the entrance; they were former patients of his. He asked them why they were there. They replied that they'd heard that there was going to be another attempt on his life that day, and they'd come to protect him. He found it amusing that little slips of girls without any weapons had come to guard him – I found it extremely moving. I still do.

The Last Guardians

For over 800 years, the prophet's burial chamber in Medina has been guarded and maintained by Abyssinian eunuchs. A few years ago, the Saudi Ministry of Islamic Affairs decreed that those currently surviving were to be the last ones, now only a handful of elderly individuals remain. They were considered devout, humble, and reclusive, and were greatly respected for living a simple life free of earthly desires.

Creative Impotence

I think art is sublimated libido. You can't be a eunuch priest, and you can't be a eunuch artist. – Anthony Burgess

When the author of *Clockwork Orange* suggested that

eunuchs could not be artists, he may have been wrong; he thought that creative energy was absent in those that cannot physically express libidinous desire. Without conventional outlets the energy builds up and eventually forces unusual paths through the psyche to relieve the pressure. Any "art" produced by a eunuch is going to be distorted and ugly, but it will exist nevertheless, no matter how contemptuously it is regarded. Eunuchs have also been priests in the past too, so I'd have to disagree with the well-known writer on these particular points.

Saint Bernard of Clairvaux

He thought rather a lot about the instruction to love your neighbour as yourself – those last two words get forgotten sometimes. He came up with the four degrees of love.

1. Love yourself for your own sake
2. Love God for your sake
3. Love God for God's sake
4. Love yourself for God's sake

It is said that we must love ourselves before we can love anyone else. Maybe love is confused with attachment or desire, but is perhaps more a deep knowing and respect, a profound kindness and compassion. It's small word that carries an enormous weight of meaning.

For most of my life I regarded self-love as a moral flaw, a narcissistic egotism that was exhibited by the vain and selfish. I sought to be selfless and humble but only damaged myself with a well-intentioned austerity of self-value that left me deformed and weak.

Thank You

I am very grateful to the following people for the support and encouragement that they showed in various ways as I struggled to compose this weird scrapbook – Ashley van Dyck, Carolina Parreria, Paul Dillon, Camilla Lewis, Amy McCauley, Martha Hayes, and Charlotte Seymour.

Some Films I Enjoyed (Perhaps You Might Like Some of Them Too)

A Moment of Innocence
All Quiet on the Western Front (the 1930 version)
Amelie
Apocalypse Now
Blade Runner
Broadway Danny Rose
Children of Heaven

Darkness in Tallin
Diary of a Lost Girl
Fat City
Full Moon in Paris
Gumshoe
Le Cop
Maidens in Uniform
Metropolis
Minna Tannenbaum
Nanny McPhee
Night on Earth
Rhythm Thief
Rodger Dodger
Silent Running
Smithereens
Snowcake
The Black Narcissus
The Hustler
The Lady in the Lake (the 1947 version)
The Long Goodbye
The Maltese Falcon
The Producers
The Third Man
The 39 Steps (the 1935 version)
Urga

Castration Fantasies

Some men fantasise about being castrated and a few actually go through with it, sometimes as part of a master/mistress-slave sado-masochistic relationship. There are apparently a few thousand such eunuchs in the USA. I don't empathise with such behaviour but understand and accept that people have different ideas and feelings about a lot of subjects. I feel much pain when I read about some of these fantasies though, as they glorify the very thing that has been a humiliating curse to me. I have also seen items written by women expressing fantasies about castrating men and have found this to be unhappy reading too.

Silver Fox

Some guys around my age manage to look rather cool. I've noticed that they always have a full head of hair and aren't fat. They also tend to dress stylishly and have a confident air about them too. Oh well, never mind.

Judar Pasha

Taken prisoner by slave-raiders as a child, he was later castrated. He served the Moroccan Sultan and was appointed to lead an invasion force from Marrakech that made a difficult crossing of the Sahara into what is now Mali. An attack across the desert had not been considered possible until then. Despite being vastly outnumbered, the small army possessed the advantage of gunpowder and defeated the imperial forces sent to repel them, subsequently taking the capital and trading cities, including fabled Timbuktu.

Bad Relationship

I haven't had a relationship with a woman since I was castrated. I wasn't a fit person to have a relationship with because I was too busy having a horrible and hateful relationship with myself. It took far too long for me to realise the full gravity of the situation. I regret that it is too late for me now.

Young Love

A boy and a girl walk along Portland Street, they are having a good-natured dispute. She vainly struggles to summon the mildest indignation about something or other but cannot maintain any resolve against his gentle teasing. He laughs tenderly as he bends down and kisses her on the cheek; she smiles ecstatically. I feel a pale happiness rise within me as I watch them pass.

Lonely

Apparently, there are two million men in our country who have no friends at all. It seems possible that men are more likely to become isolated than women; they are an invisible army made up of the defeated and the broken. When I used to call a 'phone sex service, I talked a few times with a student from London – she told me that before working on the service she had not had any idea just how many lonely men there were out there.

Body Image

I had an item published in *The Guardian*'s "My Life in Sex" series. Some of the most interesting comments posted on the website in response to the piece contained stories about other people and their situations. One lady explained that her husband had both of his testicles removed and had experienced issues relating to masculinity afterwards. Two other posters mentioned female friends who had double mastectomies, and the negative effect that this had upon them. Neither felt like a woman after the surgery, and both became shadows of their previous selves.

I had two small organs removed; logic might suggest that this wasn't such a big deal, but people aren't always rational, are they?

Materialist Mantra

Work-buy-consume-die...work-buy-consume-die... work-buy-consume-die...

It's the Way It's Done That Matters Most of All

It's a mystery to me; I know it when I see and hear it, but I don't really know how it happens. The same collection of simple chords that sound stale and uninspiring when played by many people can become full of beauty and magic in the hands of certain others. They have the gift, though even they don't know where it has come from – they were born lucky perhaps. If they try and become too clever and allow this gift that they possess to corrupt them, if they become conceited and arrogant, then they risk losing it forever.

I have been picking and strumming guitar strings since I was a teenager. I play those same simple chords, the primary colours of sound, and am enchanted by them – but I never had the magic and know I never will.

An Anonymous Label

I love music of all kinds, as long as it's good. Some very beautiful music is made by those who will never be stars, and who have an odd or unusual approach to creativity. For a few years, before the internet tsunami destroyed all in its path, I would buy obscure vinyl records on tiny little labels that no-one had heard of. You'd receive photocopied flyers with records or fanzines and there'd be addresses to order unheard wonders from. You wrote a letter and sent cash or cheque, often to some faraway place, such as the US, Japan, or Sweden. Somewhere you'd never visit. The records would arrive sometime later, and you'd place them carefully upon your turntable with anticipation. Sometimes the music was derivative and uninspiring, other times it was clumsy, awkward and completely wonderful.

One day I was sitting in my kitchen, watching the kettle whilst it came to the boil. I decided that I would set up my own little record label too; it would be a labour of love – which was just as well, as each release lost quite a lot of money. Some of these received airplay in France and Portugal, as well as in New York City, and perhaps Germany too. John Peel played one of my releases a few times. There were reviews in fanzines and music magazines which I treasured. I refused to have a website, which was obstinately stupid of course. For someone who is a bit insecure and withdrawn, lacking self-confidence, such an enterprise may not the wisest one to embark upon as you need to be a bit pushy to make things happen. Paying for records to be pressed is one thing, getting people interested in them is another matter entirely. I think I've kept every letter that came with an order and made a point of writing a friendly reply to anyone who sent an enquiry. You've probably never heard of any of the bands that I put out. I would have liked to have done better for them, been more business-like and ambitious on their behalf, but that's what major labels are for I suppose.

One day, long ago, I popped into Piccadilly Records and flicked through the racks in the Indie section. I was astounded to see one of my releases sitting there amongst records by cool and well-known bands. I wanted to say to the other patrons – "Look, I put this record out!" Naturally I contained my excitement, but it was a lovely surprise.

The label was a crazy enterprise that could only ever

fail. I'm glad that I did it though. I'd undergone my surgery a few years before and was looking for something good and positive in my life. I sought to do something creative whilst having no creative abilities of my own. I wanted to become involved, yet keep a safe distance. Music really is the food of love; I just wish I'd been a better cook.

Wei Zhongxian

He was perhaps the most feared eunuch in Chinese history. He entered service in the palace during the Ming dynasty as an attendant to Lady Wang, mother of Zhu Youjiao – who would later become Emperor. The eunuch became close to Madame Ke, who was the future Emperor's wet nurse, and the young boy became emotionally dependent upon these two individuals whom he came to consider as parents. The boy was made Emperor at fifteen. Some historians suggest that he may have had learning difficulties. He was illiterate, and uninterested in matters of state, but was a gifted carpenter who spent his time on creative projects. This permitted Wei Zhongxian to become the *de facto* ruler of the empire and issue edicts in the Emperor's name. The Donglin faction, consisting of activist scholars who sought rule based upon Confucian principles, opposed him. He assumed control of the secret police and ruthlessly purged any resistance, torturing and executing many individuals, and closing Donglin academies. His reign was cut short when the Emperor died suddenly aged twenty one, and he was ordered into exile by the new Emperor. This was not enough for his many enemies, who clamoured for a harsher penalty. Palace advisors also suggested that he was a danger whilst still alive, as he might start a rebellion. The Emperor sent soldiers to retrieve Wei Zhongian and bring him back to the capital, but whilst being transported there he hung himself with his belt.

Tales of the City

We are the stories that we tell ourselves and each other. They are places for our hearts to call home. Mythology and real life are sometimes much the same thing.

Too Nice (Note to Self)

Being "too nice" is not an excess of kindness but a lack of self-respect, which causes a desperation for approval and validation. You become a servant to other people because you lack self-worth. You make yourself a door mat and will be walked all over by people who will only have contempt for you – that's not going to enhance your value very much. You're always apologising – just another sign of your lack of self-regard. Maybe you subconsciously feel guilty about something and don't like yourself very much. Perhaps your ego requires the constant reassurance of knowing what a great job you're doing, causing you to desperately seek everyone's approval. You run around doing things for other people and neglect yourself, you get taken for granted, and you end up being resentful for all the wasted time and unappreciated effort. Living for other people's whims and needs is a good way of ignoring your own emptiness and pretending that everything is fine – everything's not fine though, is it. You're frightened of being rejected so you become too eager to please – you avoid confrontation and conflict and become a complete push-over. You go along with what other people want, and keep your views to yourself, diminishing yourself even more. Excessive empathy for others is an effective way to avoid dealing with your own issues. You'll also attract selfish and damaging personalities that will only use you and cause you harm. You'll make excuses for them and they'll become increasingly disdainful of you because of this. You end up blaming yourself for other people's faults and failings. This is no way to go through life.

A Thousand Paper Cranes

Sadako Sasaki was two years old when a nuclear bomb exploded over her hometown, Hiroshima. She was thrown through a window by the blast, and her mother carried her in her arms as she ran through the black rain of radioactive fallout, trying to escape. Nine years later she began exhibiting symptoms of acute leukaemia and was not expected to live much longer. An older girl in hospital told Sadako of the Japanese legend that if someone folds a thousand paper cranes, they are granted a wish. Even though paper was in short supply, Sadako began making origami models of this bird. There is a book which contains the suggestion that she died before achieving her task, but her family and schoolmates say that she made well over a thousand. It is also said that as she was nearing death, she held one of the paper birds in her hand and murmured – "I will write *Peace* upon your wings and you shall fly all over the world".

Sima Qian

He wrote a famous history of China over two thousand years ago – *Records of the Grand Historian*. This was written in a jizhuanti style; a form of narrative that predominantly employs biographies and is not necessarily linear. This monumental work is regarded as being one of the foundational texts of Chinese civilisation and greatly influenced subsequent written histories in China and other Asian countries.

Sima Qian was a court official who spoke up for a disgraced military officer and was sentenced to death for this. His sentence was commuted to castration or the payment of a large sum of money. As he was not wealthy, he was subjected to the first of these and then imprisoned for three years. Upon his release he refused to commit suicide, as was expected of a scholar who had been disgraced with castration. He lived in the imperial palace as a eunuch, where he completed the great work for which he is still known.

Romantic Idealisation

Of all the manifestations of the universe, none is greater than woman. The Book of Genesis suggests that God stopped all creation activities once woman had been made; there was no further to go, the ultimate master-work had been achieved. It is also sometimes the case that women can be the biggest pain in the backside in the entire universe too – but even that's just part of what makes them so wonderful.

Self-Pity

An occasional wallow in this delicious indulgence is quite natural, can perhaps even be a positive thing, but when it becomes a habit it's very harmful. Feeling sorry for yourself might sometimes be a therapeutic response to a difficulty or a traumatic event, but it is only a healthy part of a healing process if taken in small amounts, very sparingly. Overdosing is destructive, then becomes an emotional narcotic, where suffering disguises itself as a pleasure and opportunities for real happiness are spurned. The addict revels in failure, delights in fear, and enjoys self-inflicted agony.

Self-pity is an inverted form of validation. Your perceived value increases in proportion to the supposed unfairness of your lot. The more hopeless your situation, the more noble your suffering. You nurture your pain, preventing healing so that you can enjoy the exquisite misery that you crave and eventually come to depend on. You manufacture a completely false sense of value by creating a series of grievances and injustices which you recite regularly. These give you all the excuses you need for failure, and a reason not to try in the first place, but you're only degrading and harming yourself.

Personality (I Wish I Had One)

Apparently, I am an INFP (Introversion, iNtuition, Feeling, Perception) on the Myers-Briggs Type Indicator; though such classifications can only ever be general ones as everyone is a unique individual. Amongst other characteristics, INFPs are driven by a strong sense of right and wrong and a desire to encourage creativity around them, even if just in behind-the-scenes roles. Their weaknesses include sensitivity to criticism, poor organisation, and low assertiveness. They are idealists who may appear reserved or shy but have passions hidden deep within them; they are often misunderstood by other people. INFPs have a tendency to become lost in contemplation and lose touch with reality, withdrawing into themselves and making it hard for others to connect with them sometimes. They are intuitive and altruistic, generally avoiding conflict but prepared to stand up fiercely for their values when necessary.

The Chotto Matte Man

Chotto matte, in Japanese, means – "Hold on, wait" – the softly spoken message that Yukio Shige has for tormented souls standing on the Tonjinbo cliffs, a well-known beauty spot, and a place where people come to commit suicide. He was a police officer stationed nearby and was struck by the number of times that he helped retrieve bodies from the bottom of the cliffs. He was surprised that nobody tried to prevent this tragic procession. Once he'd retired, he began patrolling the area, keeping an eye out for solitary individuals standing silently by themselves, looking out to sea. He would approach them and ask – "Are you okay?" He would listen, and then suggest that there were other ways to deal with their problems, that someone would help them. He now has a team of volunteers assisting him as part of a non-profit organisation that owns a cafe nearby and has apartments where those who have turned back from the brink may stay for a while if they've nowhere else to go. The team have prevented several hundred suicides over the years.

He was motivated to begin his work when he encountered an old couple sitting near the cliffs, just before he retired from the police. Their business had failed, and they had come to throw themselves off the cliffs at sunset. He convinced them not to do this and called a patrol car to take them to the local welfare bureau. Five days later he received a letter from them, written just before they had hung themselves, thanking him for his kindness. He was outraged by the indifference that the couple had been shown by the authorities and vowed to do something for those who saw no other option than ending their lives. When people come to the cliffs with an intention to end their suffering, they don't immediately jump. They stand or sit by themselves for hours, looking out to sea, thinking. They do not really want to kill themselves but have no-one to talk to. The volunteers encourage troubled people to come with them to the cafe, where they are given tea and cake, and treated with kindness and respect. The cafe is run by Misako Kawagoshi, who lost both her parents to suicide when she was a child. She herself has contemplated suicide in the past too and says that she feels that she is looking at herself when she sees the people standing at the cliffs.

Many who were convinced by the team not to jump have kept in touch and come back to visit regularly, grateful that Mr Shige and his volunteers took the time to listen and help.

Angels

Some have suggested that the Christian concept of angels shares specific characteristics with those of eunuchs – tall, beardless, non-sexual beings with beautiful voices. In the tenth century, the imperial court of Byzantium was held to be an earthly replica of heaven, with the Emperor fulfilling the role of deity and the attendant eunuchs that of angels.

Stanislav Petrov

On the 26th September 1983, Stanislav Petrov was the duty officer at the Soviet Union's early warning command centre in Oko. He received an alert that the US had launched five nuclear missiles, and protocol dictated that he call his superiors in Moscow so that a retaliatory strike could be ordered. He decided to ignore protocol and use his common sense instead. He reasoned that if the US was going to initiate a nuclear conflict, it would have launched a large number of missiles to inflict devastating blows upon the Soviet Union. He sat thinking silently whilst alarms went off and eventually decided to report a fault in the computer system instead – he made the correct decision. A flaw in the system had led to satellites mistaking the reflected glare of sunlight for exhaust flares of incoming missiles. The system was new, and Petrov had little faith in it; he later said that people were wiser than computers. He was also the only officer in the team that had received a civilian education and was therefore prepared to question any information that he received. He was reprimanded for not recording the incident in accordance with documentation protocols and re-assigned to a less responsible role. He later took early retirement. One day Stanislav Petrov broke the rules and saved the world from a possible nuclear war. It's perhaps fortunate for all of us that it was him that was on duty that particular day.

Mughal Eunuchs

The Indian Mughals employed eunuchs in their seraglios and harems for several centuries. Amongst other roles, eunuchs guarded the Emperor and shared this duty with female soldiers called Urdubegis. European visitors found the eunuchs to be particularly insolent. Niccolao Manucci travelled to, and worked in, the imperial court and noted their "licentious tongues". He also wrote – "another of their qualities is to be friendly to women and inimical to men, which may be from envy, knowing what they've been deprived of." Often, eunuchs were kidnapped whilst young, or sold into slavery by their parents as boys, then castrated. Manucci relates that one senior eunuch was surprised to receive an elderly couple from Bengal, who claimed to be his parents. He ordered them to receive fifty lashes each for having the temerity to visit him after "having been the cause, by emasculating me, of depriving me of the greatest pleasures attainable in this world".

Some Characteristics of Introverts

Find social situations to be emotionally draining
Enjoy solitude
Difficult to get to know as they don't open up easily
Prefer to learn by observing

Can feel more alone in a crowd than when they are on their own

Feel like a fake when networking or meeting new people

Dislike being the centre of attention

Don't need much from other people

Notice tiny details

Feel at home in the world of thoughts

Like to "people watch"

Good listeners

Small circle of friends

Prefer to have meaningful conversations than empty chit-chat

Spend a lot of time pondering

Don't know what to say sometimes

Have a "public self" and a "private self" which are very different from each other

Will often mentally rehearse what they're going to say before speaking

Tendency to bottle up emotions

Better at writing thoughts than speaking them

Not very concerned with wealth and status

Can concentrate on something for long periods

Risk averse

Likely to let calls go to voicemail

Tend to put off making decisions

Tasteless

Research indicates that obese people have a reduced sense of taste in comparison to normal people. I've noted that "foodies", who enthuse at great length about subtleties of various dishes, are often rather thin. Fatties like me joylessly shovel in great quantities of junk and don't really notice flavours unless they're particularly strong or sweet.

Eunuch Porn

A niche category; often a sub-genre of CBT (Cock and Ball Torture) and BDSM (Bondage/Discipline, Domination/Submission, and Sado-Masochism). Also features in some humiliation and cuckolding fantasies – none of which appeal to me really.

Pomona

The apartments were going to be built, the wild and discarded island was about to become a construction site, and barriers had been put up. I found that I could walk outside the rail overlooking the ship canal and around the fence. Later, even this route was closed off once the site had been fully secured. Something had to be done, so I'd placed an order that had arrived a few days later, and here I was.

I'd heard that ships came to Pomona from far flung places once, when the docks had been operating, and sometimes when their cargoes were unloaded exotic seeds had spilled out. These had lain dormant in the soil for years before occasionally germinating and pushing up oddly incongruous blooms into the Manchester sky. I'd also read about people seed-bombing building sites and thought this a wonderfully noble action.

The Atacama is one of the driest regions in the world. One spring it experienced the heaviest rains for years due to the El Niño weather pattern. The land was covered in an expanse of desert flowers which normally only bloom sporadically at intervals of several years. Pink, purple and white covered the normally drab landscape, attracting butterflies. In Death Valley the same phenomenon led to a brief and intense explosion of yellow.

I sowed as I walked, one dull afternoon, sprinkling and scattering seeds over the newly turned soil. I laid a secret carpet of hope, watched by an occasional disinterested tram passenger. I'm certain that my gesture was futile but, oddly, this made it more necessary. One day the rains may come. Who can say? The desert might bloom.

I planted wildflower seeds – twenty thousand meadow buttercup, ten thousand red campion, seven thousand red clover and five thousand cornflower. I wonder if any of them will ever flower.

Oh Well

Should I revel in my brokenness, celebrate my distortedness? Perhaps I need only to accept the way things are and not allow myself to be beaten by them every day, I have been fighting myself in a pointless conflict that has caused me great damage.

I did my best with what I had available at the time. If I had been better equipped I would have navigated out of the darkness a long time ago. But it wasn't to be. There is no point in beating myself up about it anymore. I suppose I have reached a point where I can offer a form of forgiveness to myself; for being what I am and for doing what I did to myself.

The Henry Watson Music Library

The music library is on the first floor in Manchester Central Library. It's named after Dr Henry Watson, who worked as an errand boy in a music shop and taught himself to play a variety of instruments. Once he had become successful, he founded the library so that others could learn music without the difficulties he had encountered.

Sometimes there's a beautiful cacophony of various instruments playing different pieces simultaneously. Teachers give lessons on hired pianos here.

One day I walked in and was met with the most wonderful music; it stopped me on the spot. It was a magically unfamiliar piece being played beautifully. Other people had stopped what they were doing, their heads raised, held by a spell that moved through the air. I carefully approached the source and saw a girl in red sitting at one of the pianos, her hands dancing over the keyboard, her body swaying with the energy of the music that she was creating.

A young guy in a bobble hat plays something unknown and lovely; a few mistakes and hesitations make it more beautiful than bland technical proficiency would.

A girl plays a piano, very well. Then another girl arrives, and a lesson commences – the new arrival is a beginner. The teacher patiently leads her through a piece several times and they speak in a language that I am unable to identify – something European, I think. I hear the teacher say – "*Unu, doi, zei, patru*" a few times. Sometimes when you listen to people speak a language that you don't understand it is like listening to music. After the pupil left on completion of the lesson, and whilst the teacher was waiting for someone else to arrive, I approached her. She told me that she'd been speaking Romanian; I had little idea that it could sound so lovely.

'Mood Indigo' is haltingly picked out on a piano, a pleasant surprise. I commend the player upon his choice; he suggests that he needs to practice it a bit more.

One day I listened to a lunchtime performance of one of Schnittke's piano works at the RNCM, then in the early evening saw the performer giving a lesson here. She was a fourth-year student; I told her how much I had enjoyed hearing her play earlier.

An elderly chap comes sometimes; he wears a suit and sits at a piano. I'm always glad when I see him. Whilst he plays, he is somewhere else, a place unreachable without a musical ticket for the journey there. Another older guy wearing corduroy trousers and a woolly hat often picks expertly on a guitar as afternoons drift by.

Bald

I look like Uncle Fester from the *Addams Family* film – without the charisma and sex appeal, obviously. There's not much you can do when your hair's gone; I certainly wouldn't consider artificial replacement or a transplant. I'm not too bothered about being bald myself but realise that the way that people perceive you is often based upon your appearance. When I was a member of an online dating site, I noticed that a few women stated very emphatically that they didn't wish to hear from men who were bald.

The Indescribably Sad Palace of Pleasure

I built a pleasure palace in my head; first I constructed a framework of synthetic desire, and then wrapped it with neural pathways that lit up when connected to the mains. I decorated my hidden retreat with myths and fantasies, and holograms of beautiful girls. I tried to pretend that it wasn't plastic; sometimes I almost managed to convince myself. I wound ever more strings of neon around my little den, like a homeowner who has lost all sense of proportion as Christmas approaches, and who drapes their house in an excess of tastelessness. I made this haven of artificial brightness to illuminate the darkness that I had taken refuge in to escape from the brightness outside that I no longer belonged to. I attempted to convince myself that I had made a galaxy of stars, which cast an intense glow that I danced in by myself. It was the only place where I thought I could truly be myself, but I never discovered who that was, maybe there is no me really. When I visited my secret pleasure palace, I imagined that I was out there, in the bright sunlight, but I wasn't really. I was only fooling myself that I was having fun, that I was alive, that it was real. I couldn't maintain the illusion, but how I tried. My little pleasure palace is the saddest and loneliest place that I have ever known.

Avoiding the Subject

George Carter Stent visited imperial China in the late nineteenth century and later wrote about his experiences. He was permitted admittance to the imperial court and observed eunuchs there. He noted that people would avoid reference to broken objects in the presence of eunuchs so as not to insult them, but also permitted increased latitude in their behaviour. He recorded that – "A great freedom of speech and manner is allowed to eunuchs, on account of their deprivation; manner and conduct that would not be tolerated in others being overlooked in them with the remark – 'he is only a eunuch'."

Fig + Sparrow

It's a small haven on Oldham Street with wooden floors and tables, a high ceiling, and a pleasant atmosphere. In the nook next to the counter there were two loose wooden panels in the wall; behind these were contained a constantly growing collection of messages scribbled upon receipts and pages torn from notebooks. They might be described as being philosophical in nature. The original one was written in green ink and said…

Dear fellow discoverer,

We are so happy that you found this note.
   This afternoon my brother and I have been chatting about life, and where we're at, where we thought we'd be at this point.
   We just wanted to let you know that wherever you're at, and whatever you're doing in life at the moment,
   You are ok, you're doing great.
   Keep going.

There were well over twenty messages there once, before the panels fell out. I left a note there too – the fourth one, it had a date and my name upon it. I tried to think of something pithy yet profound but wasn't quite able to manage this.

The Colour

The Galli of Ancient Rome wore yellow whilst conducting their celebrations of emasculation, and the Eunuch's Battalion of the Ming dynasty wore yellow armour to distinguish them from other soldiers. In our culture, it is traditionally associated with cowardice, which is often interpreted as a lack of manliness and masculine virtues such as courage and resilience, mettle and fortitude.

Black Noise

In fields such as audio engineering, colours are some-times assigned to describe the power spectrum of vari-ous noise signals. Most people will have heard of White Noise; there are many others – Pink, Brown, Blue etc. The colour is usually assigned by comparison of the spec-tra emitted by noise and light. Black Noise is perceived as silence, and sometimes it is just that – an absence of sound. At other times though, it contains noise signals which are outside the frequencies that are discernible to the human ear, but still affect the environment that they're part of. Silence isn't always so quiet perhaps.

If the city were to stop, even for a second, it would die. It never does though. It lives in invisible poems and textured sounds, always different but always the same. It is singing to us, but we don't listen. Just close your eyes, let the pictures and images blur together, don't try and catch any of them, allow them to flow freely. Do you want to know a secret? Anyone can discover it, but most don't think to try; it's obscured by being so obvious. You might have to practice a little – don't listen too hard or you won't hear.

There

      yes, there

            the silent music

                  it's beautiful, isn't it?

Mockery

It's human nature – you have to be prepared to deal with it. It still hurts of course. Men incline towards a more straightforward brutality but perhaps also sense within themselves a deep fear of castration when they laugh at me. Ladies tend to be more subtle, and much more hurtful. I have never retaliated or shown any reaction to unkind humour, and perhaps it would have been healthier for me emotionally had I stood up for myself a bit more. Such scorn is a comparatively rare occurrence as most people aren't aware of what I am; it's my shameful little secret. When I was first castrated, I was determined to just get on with life and be open about what had happened. I wasn't strong enough to maintain this resolve and retreated into my shell like a craven mollusc when unpleasant humour was directed towards me.

Coward

It is one of the greatest humiliations in the masculine lexicon – a woman can never be a coward. Everyone feels fear, it's natural, but this remains largely unacknowledged because it is a shameful thing to admit to. There is a special contempt reserved for men who have been overwhelmed by fear; they are the objects of a particularly bitter scorn. Often, it is a specific event that exposes a deep-rooted flaw that may have escaped previous notice.

Fleeing fear is exhausting, eventually a moment may come when you are too tired to run any further. Finally, you stand and face the foe that has hunted you down relentlessly, you give yourself up to annihilation. But it doesn't move in to kill you because it can't, it's not really there, it never was. It's a hologram that can itself have no effect, but by influencing your thoughts it gains great power. In fact, if you walk towards it with open arms it will disappear. Fear diminishes when embraced with kindness and craves its own destruction. It will demand that you destroy it with increasing desperation until you comply, or it has paralysed you. Fear is personal, as it is a product of each individual's psyche. The fear of suffering was itself what caused so much suffering in my life. By trying to avoid pain I lost opportunities for happiness. It takes courage to be happy sometimes, and I was too scared to be able to fully experience happiness. I was oppressed by a fear that I did not really perceive or understand; I retreated into a small darkness within myself and hid there. The only mitigation that I can allow is that I was unaware of so many things – including how to truly be myself, and how to deal with the situation I found myself in.

Puddles

For a city that is celebrated for rainfall, Manchester does not appear to have a particularly efficient drainage system. It would probably cost rather a lot of money and require a civil commitment that is beyond our current culture to remedy this. When it rains heavily, enormous black puddles appear in certain streets. They ripple as cyclists pass through them, and cold dirty water is splashed over pedestrians when indifferent cars ford these small lakes at speed. Sometimes the clouds pass, and light reflects off these wet mirrors and, where the urban geography is favourable, dismal streets are brightened by reflected illumination. I mapped some of the more remarkable examples on my wanderings. If you look carefully into these windows to a parallel universe, you may see another city that appears similar to this one but is actually very different. You may occasionally notice a rainbow reflected in one of these puddles, but when you look up there isn't one in the sky above. These temporary apertures show us the city as it could be, if our better natures prevailed. A place made up of hopes that have struggled vainly against reality and been extinguished, yet live forever in the city of dreams that may be glimpsed briefly in the temporary looking glasses created on fortunate rainy days.

Some Good Books I Read

A Confederacy of Dunces – John Kennedy Toole
A Mind of Its Own – Cordelia Fine
A Philosophy of Walking – Frederic Gros
All Quiet on the Western Front – Erich Maria
    Remarque
Bliss and Other Stories – Katherine Mansfield
Celebrating Life – Jonathan Sacks
Chattering – Louise Stern
Chernobyl – Serhii Plokhy
Childless Voices – Lorna Gibb
Chocolate Nations – Orla Ryan
Collected Stories – VS Pritchett
Devil Girls – Ed Wood Jr
Ground Control – Anna Minton
Hackney, That Rose Red Empire – Iain Sinclair
I Choose Elena – Lucia Osborne-Crowley
I Shall Not Hate – Izzeldin Abuelaish
If Nobody Speaks of Remarkable Things – Jon
    McGregor
Ishmael – Daniel Quinn
Kitchen – Banana Yoshimoto
Kolyma Tales – Varlam Shalamov
Leave It to Psmith – PG Wodehouse
Like Water for Chocolate – Laura Esqivel
Love and Garbage – Ivan Klima
Momo – Michael Ende

My Face for the World to See – Candy Darling
My Fellow Prisoners – Mikhail Khodorkovsky
Night Haunts – Sukhdev Sandhu
One Flew Over the Cuckoo's Nest – Ken Kesey
Riot Days – Maria Alyokhina
Small Acts of Resistance – Steve Crawshaw & Steve Jackson
Sophie's World – Jostein Gaarder
Sorry I'm Late, I Didn't Want to Come – Jessica Pan
Sweden's Dark Soul – Kajsa Norman
Tao Te Ching – Lao Tzu
The Angel of Grozny – Asne Seierstad
The Beekeeper of Sinjar – Dunya Mikhail
The Chains of Heaven – Philip Marsden
The Endless Steppe – Esther Hautzig
The Examined Life – Stephen Grosz
The Great Gatsby – F Scott Fitzgerald
The Guest Cat – Takashi Hiraide
The Heart and the Bottle – Oliver Jeffers
The Heart is a Lonely Hunter – Carson McCullers
The Illustrated Man – Ray Bradbury
The Innocent Libertine – Colette
The Maltese Falcon – Dashiel Hammett
The Man Who Fell to Earth – Walter Tevis
The Philosophy of Andy Warhol – Pat Hackett & Andy Warhol
The Power and the Glory – Graham Greene

Roll the Credits

I think that those who put in the behind-the-scenes effort that goes into the publication of a book should get a bit more recognition sometimes. So, I ask you to join me in a moment of appreciation and applause for the following –

Hannah Bourne-Taylor ....prologue editor
Johanna Craven.........................proof-reader
Cait Gabe-Jones ....copy-editor
Felicity Hall..............................proof-reader
Tom Perrin ....publisher

The Wonder Inn

I'd been there for a gig and was later involved with the Lost & Found Museum exhibition. I began helping out there, doing some unpaid voluntary work. It was a project unlike anything else I had ever been involved with. It lived in a rundown building right in town, on the edge of the Northern Quarter, which had been a number of different things over the years – a grain and wheat store, a tobacco warehouse, a tailor's workshop, a wholesale store. There are three floors – the top one was an artist's space where some wonderful work was created. The middle floor had a large space, the Ballroom, for events, and a smaller area known as the Garden Room, which contained a lot of plants and also had a wide range of uses. There'd be yoga, martial arts, music gigs, exhibitions, early morning non-alcoholic dance raves and comedy nights held there. There were also wedding receptions and wakes, and a lot of other unusual goings-on. Downstairs had a bar and vegan café, as well as a couple more spaces that were used for events such as those mentioned above. I just helped out; lugged furniture around, assisted setting up for events and cleaned up afterwards.

The Wonder Inn was a quirky, bohemian splash upon the grimy consumerism of its surroundings. I was a bit of an anomaly I suppose; everyone there was young and creative whilst I'm an old square, but I derived a great sense of purpose from being involved. It was a pleasure to see so many wonderful people passing through with each event. Every day I went in it was like the fairies had come in during the night and moved everything about. There was always something going on there. It's gone now, sadly, but it is still in my heart.

A Twisted Identity

Augustine of Hippo said that castrated eunuchs were – "neither changed into a woman nor allowed to remain a man". I still mostly think like a heterosexual male, even though I'm neutered and impotent.

Eunuch is a pejorative term, its utterance an eternal insult. It is a name that expresses disempowerment, disfigurement, and diminishment. Eunuchs are emasculated but not feminised; most are chemically or surgically castrated for medical reasons and did not wish for this to have occurred to them. Some males seek castration however, sometimes as a transition stage towards becoming female, sometimes for various other reasons.

Gender is sometimes nowadays seen as being a spectrum, rather than a binary definition. Even with so many options for gender identity available there are still some who do not have a place to call home. Eunuchs are reluctant to draw attention to themselves; they fear shame and humiliation, wish to evade the contempt and scorn that is their eternal burden. They lurk in the shadows, hoping that they will not be discovered. Yet they still wish to walk in the light, as all living beings must, no matter how despised and lowly they may be.

Radio Argot

It was a tiny record label that released four very limited one-sided 12" records in screen-printed sleeves. It was the project of Gabby Warshawer, who sold candy bars on the New York subway to fund the first release whilst she was still at high school. About ten years ago I somehow tracked her down and conducted a short e-mail interview that I intended to include in a 'zine that I never got around to finishing. Gabby published a 'zine about indie-pop called Double Whammy with a schoolfriend in the mid-1990s, and also held roof-top gigs at her parent's apartment block in mid-town Manhattan. Extension cables were lowered to a window on the third floor and plugged in to power the amplifiers and equipment. Small groups played there amongst the surrounding skyscrapers – boy/girl duos Kumari, I Live The Life Of A Movie Star Secret Hideout, and The Poconos. The label, 'zine and gigs only lasted until Gabby went to college and began new chapters in her life.

Making a Pass

I met some friends at a restaurant in town for lunch. The waitress was very nice, about forty perhaps, far too young for me. I knew I had no chance, so this gave me the courage to ask her if she'd like to meet me for a drink. She replied that she was married but thanked me for my invitation all the same. It was the first time I'd made a pass at a woman in over two decades, I was really nervous, but she was very nice about it, I'll always be grateful to her for that.

Some Suicidal Symptoms

Helplessness
Hopelessness
Social Withdrawal
Loss of enthusiasm for life

Hermotimus

He was a Persian eunuch who came to be favoured by Xerxes the Great during the wars against Greece of 480 BC. Once he had achieved the power of the King's favour, he is said to have extracted revenge upon the man who had castrated him as a boy – Panionius. He forced him to castrate his sons under threat of death, then ordered the sons to castrate their father.

Young Love

A couple stand outside the Koffee Pot, looking at the menu. A petite pretty girl, and a tall sweet boy with a mop of unbrushed hair. They hold hands as they discuss possible choices. She pulls his arm to get his attention, he must kiss her right now – immediately. He complies willingly, his long body bends whilst she stretches up onto her toes. They just can't get enough of each other; I smile and remember when I could feel that way too.

Devastation

I strolled around the Northern Quarter one summer evening but was stopped in my tracks when a girl walked past. It was like being hit by a truck; I thought she was jaw-droppingly gorgeous whilst also being completely ordinary at the same time. She wore a colourfully striped top – a sleeveless rainbow. I watched her disappear around a corner with awestruck admiration. A few minutes later and…there she was again! She'd looped back with a friend; they were looking for somewhere to eat and studied the menu beside a doorway. After a moment they decided to go somewhere else and headed off. She was gone, for good this time, leaving me crumpled in her wake. There were lots of other good-looking girls about town that evening, but this one had rendered them invisible; some women have the ability to do that.

I thought about her all the way home, she stirred me up terribly. I glumly sat with my guitar and sang a sad song very badly. Then I burst into tears and wept uncontrollably; all the shame, loneliness and despair surging up from deep within me. How pathetic; a fat, repulsive old eunuch destroyed by a pretty young woman.

Note to Self

Stupid…worthless…piece of shit (repeat endlessly)

Mohamed Khan Qajar

He was captured by a rival ruling family as a child; instead of being killed, the boy was castrated and released. It was an unsettled era in what is now Iran, with several ruling families fighting over what had been a great empire that was disintegrating into unstable fiefdoms. He was a cruel ruler, dealing with defeated foes in the harshest manner. He was also an effective military leader and an adept politician. He reunited the former empire after several years of campaigning that cost many lives and had the title Shahanshah – King of Kings – bestowed upon him. He's also noted for moving the capital from Shiraz to Tehran, where it has remained ever since.

Viking Raiders

It has been suggested that amongst several reasons for the Vikings attacking monasteries in the British Isles during the early Middle Ages was to provide eunuchs for the Byzantine and Abbasid empires. Literate boys and men were captured and sold to slave-traders, then taken to Venice, where they were castrated. They were then sold on for a considerable profit, feeding a demand for educated castrates.

Banal Reflections Discovered in a Dog-Eared Notebook

Ravel observed that the orchestra has the capacity to destroy the material that it plays. So, it is with writing; the way words are used can degrade their meaning.

Desire is limitless whilst objects of desire are finite – craving cannot ever be satisfied.

We seek pleasure in the mistaken belief that it will

make us happy, it won't – happiness and pleasure are two very different places.

The various ways that different qualities of light touches things; air, land, water, people – is quite astounding.

God is not a concept that we have invented. God is the deepest expression of us and our true being.

Sport is like sex; it's more fun being a participant than a spectator.

Democratic Delusions

A lot of people seem to enjoy working themselves into a rage about politicians; it's practically a national sport nowadays. Politicians have little real power; we are all just servants of capitalism. John F. Kennedy, or perhaps more likely Ted Sorensen, his advisor, said that people get the politicians that they deserve. Voters prefer politicians who say what the voters wish to hear. The people want politicians to make impossible promises that the people themselves know can never be delivered. The electorate doesn't want to hear any truths, they want delicious lies instead. Then they want to abuse politicians for telling them what they wanted to hear, for being a true reflection of what they are themselves. The politicians that best express the mood of the people are the ones that are successful and get elected, so they can't afford to tell the truth. They have to give people the comforting fantasies they seek, or they will be rejected. Our politicians are just fine actually; it's the general population that needs to change.

The Day Everything Stopped

The pressure increased continuously over a long time; cracks began to appear. The darkness inside me grew ceaselessly until one day it overwhelmed me. I could still breathe and walk but had become completely disconnected from myself, the world, and everyone in it. I felt as though I was an empty shadow, and nothing was real. Everything was an illusion. Even though I could see people and converse with them, I perceived that they were just holograms, and that I was too. My new displaced perspective allowed me to see the pixels on the screen, the hidden props that held the backdrops in position, the terrifying fakeness of *everything*. I understood then that life was a virtual reality experience, a game played on the biggest console. I had taken a wrong turning and was walking around behind the scenery, had arrived somewhere that I was not supposed to, an unintended visitor. I didn't know how I'd got there, or how to leave. I was totally, indescribably…lost.

We All Sing Unheard Love Songs

The US Navy deploys sonar and hydroponic listening equipment in the Pacific Ocean to detect and track submarines. In the early 1990s it began picking up a weird signal that baffled the military experts, nothing similar had been heard before. Eventually the oceanography institute at Woods Hole in Massachusetts suggested that it was most probably a blue whale. The dates and location of recorded detections correlated with the migratory path of this species. Both sexes of the blue whale can vocalise, but it's generally the males that sing when attempting to attract a mate. The odd thing was that this one was singing at the "wrong" frequency; 10 to 39 hertz is the normal range for blue whale song but this one sung at 52 hertz – a much higher pitch. The pattern of his call was different too – shorter and more frequent, with variations. It seemed that he travelled alone, as other whale song was never detected in the same vicinity as his. The press developed the story and christened him "the loneliest whale in the world", condemned to wander the ocean singing unheeded, although there's no evidence that other whales couldn't hear his unusual call. Plenty of theories have been offered, unsuccessful searches have been conducted, but Blue 52 has never been found. Actually, he hasn't been heard from for a few years either. What caused him to become silent?

Repressed Emotions

The most dangerous aspect of repression is its unconscious nature; you don't realise what you're doing to yourself. Whilst you may sometimes knowingly suppress feelings for good reason, repression is a hidden enemy that causes great damage.

Making It Happen

Often people suggest that you shouldn't try too hard searching for love – "don't go looking for it, it will come along when you least expect it". I can tell you from experience that this is not the case. I've been least expecting it for two decades and it didn't come along. Happiness and love really do not come looking for you; you've got to make these things happen yourself...if you can.

Note to Self

So, no one loves you? There must be a reason for that, see if you can work it out for yourself. Have you got it yet, Einstein?

Eunuch Writings

These are extremely scarce. Liu Ruyou was a eunuch in the imperial Chinese court in the sixteenth and seventeenth centuries, he was imprisoned until death and took the opportunity to compose memoirs which described the many comings and goings inside the palace. He noted that some eunuchs were "besotted with the fairer sex" and would be at "a woman's beck and call". Over two thousand years ago, Sima Qian wrote a letter in which he stated that there was "no defilement so great as castration", and that "one who has undergone such a punishment nowhere counts as a man". He also spoke of the shame that he felt, saying "better that I should hide in the farthest depths of the mountains". Xin Xiu Ming wrote a memoir in the early twentieth century, in which he speaks of the eunuch's lot; greatly despised and punished by their own peculiar suffering, he described the palace eunuchs as having no hope for the future and taking comfort in opium. Professor Richard Wassenburg was chemically castrated following a diagnosis of prostate cancer and has written and broadcast about his experience very eloquently. The arrival of the internet has provided opportunities for others to post messages that deal with various aspects of castration and identity. Mostly, those who are willing to express themselves have chosen to be castrated for their own various personal reasons. The majority of modern eunuchs, who did not choose emasculation, remain hidden in silent shame.

Some Good Places to Get a Tea or Coffee in Manchester

Ancoats Coffee Co
Ancoats General Store
Art of Tea
Ezra & Gil
Federal
Fig + Sparrow
Grindsmith
Idle Hands
International Anthony Burgess Foundation
Kim By The Sea
Koffee Pot
Nexus Art Cafe
North Star Piccadilly
North Tea Power
Pop Up Bikes
Pot Kettle Black
Proper Tea
Siop Shop
Takk
Teacup Kitchen
Trove Ancoats

Battlefield Castrations

It is a long-established practice of warfare to castrate defeated foes. Often this occurs as part of a wider pattern of sexual violence designed to humiliate the victims and empower the perpetrators. The castration of prisoners was carried out by ancient armies of Egypt, Persia, China and many more since. When Italian forces invaded Abyssinia in the late nineteenth century, prisoners were castrated by the victorious defenders. In the twenty-first Century the Janjaweed militia castrated civilians as part of an ethnic cleansing campaign in southern Sudan.

During the First World War, cases of castration injuries due to gunshot and shrapnel wounds were recorded. It was noted that those affected tended not only to be deprived of sexual virility and the ability to become a father, but often also appeared to lose much interest in life generally as well.

It is reported that some victims of the Bataclan attack in Paris were castrated after being taken hostage. It has also been recorded that some victims of lynch mobs in the USA were castrated before being killed.

Purple Bloom

The red rose of Lancaster is one of the floral emblems of Manchester, as is Cotton-Grass apparently. The unofficial flower of the city might well be Buddleia; it's everywhere. It can be seen growing on chimney stacks and rooftops, protruding from walls, ledges and bridges. No foothold is too slight for it to take root. When in flower it splashes purple onto the drab brick and concrete terrain of the urban desert. Its fragrance is lovely too; smell one when it's blooming, and you'll see what I mean.

Sour Grapes

When I was young, I thought most girls wanted a guy who was attentive, respectful and caring. Perhaps they do, but they also want other things that I didn't offer them. A woman wants a man who will challenge her; psychologically, and emotionally – someone who will stretch her, and take her out of her comfort zone. Unfortunately, I didn't realise this until it was too late; I was a complete softie, a big teddy bear. I was a tiresome square who tried very hard to be such a great guy but could only ever be bland and one-dimensional. I recall a girlfriend telling me with a curled lip that I was like a faithful and affectionate dog, at the time I didn't understand why this made her so angry. On another occasion a girlfriend was giving me some grief for no obvious reason, she stopped suddenly with a puzzled expression and asked me – "Why am I being so horrible to you?" I didn't know the answer then, but I do now – I wasn't doing it for her. I didn't turn her on, I didn't engage her fully. A woman wants a man who gives her an involuntary shiver deep in her heart; some guys can't do that to a woman, and never will. If she wants a dog, she'll go to the kennels and choose one. If she wants a teddy bear she'll go to the toy store and buy one. If she wants a man, she'll go to a bar and get herself picked up by one.

Kind and affectionate, sweet and considerate, patient and caring are *not* truly male characteristics and, more than anything, a woman wants a man to be a MAN.

Oh, just listen to me, I'm having a real whinge, aren't I? Yeah, life's not fair – blah, blah, blah. Poor lonely eunuch, left on the shelf, bitter and sad. Why don't I just shut up? Okay then, please forget my resentful little outburst and let's move along.

Winter Fragments

There's a cold, freezing fog, thick and heavy. Pavements are slippery, a thin layer of treachery upon them. The sunshine almost breaks through in the afternoon, but not quite. Where the light is strongest, small sparkling pieces of glitter swirl in the air; tiny ice particles catching the light – a rare and beautiful display.

Hailstones bounce hard upon the ground and a roof that is lit by the cold sun. A reassuring white noise; stop for a while and listen from a sheltered spot.

A young couple wearing woolly hats, warm gloves, and puffed down jackets. They smile happily at each other, their laughter condensing in the cold air. My heart thaws briefly as they walk past me.

Vapour trails in a pale blue sky; paths to the future, escapes routes from the past.

Cult Eunuchs

Several members of the Heaven's Gate group were found to have been castrated when autopsies were carried out on the bodies of those who had participated in a mass suicide in March 1997.

The Skoptsy were a secret sect that existed in Tsarist Russia for a couple of centuries. They were known to require that male members be castrated, and that female members undergo mastectomies, as part of "fiery baptisms". The cult was persecuted by the authorities from the late eighteenth century onwards, it is thought that they might have had close to a hundred thousand members in the early twentieth century. Their numbers rapidly declined under communism, and it is thought that this sect may now have died out completely.

There are reports that several hundred followers of the Indian guru, Gurmeet Ram Rahim Singh, have been castrated so as to be "nearer to God". This is disputed by his organisation.

The Valesians were a heretical Christian sect that existed in the Middle East in the fourth century, they advocated castration as a path to God.

Everyone Has the Whiff of Loneliness About Them

I was certain that it was a Charlie Chaplin quote, but I couldn't discover anyone who had said it. Maybe I did, in a shock display of originality. Loneliness is all around us yet is also the most shameful affliction. There is always an unspoken suggestion of blame, that loneliness is a curse caused by a perceived failing or inadequacy in those who are subject to it. It is an invisible malady that crushes many souls; we might pass many sufferers each day, unaware of their condition. I am constantly overwhelmed by its cold and empty embrace.

The First Date in Two Decades

One time when I went speed dating it led to a date; my first for twenty years in fact. I'd got a bit distracted by proceedings and had forgotten to write notes on the form provided or to tick the numbers of the ladies I thought were particularly nice. I couldn't remember which lady was which at the end of the evening when you hand the form in. I was later informed by the event organiser that one lady had ticked my number and was given her e-mail address to contact her if I wished. I did so, and she agreed to meet. I didn't know which lady she was, but she was someone prepared to meet me over a drink and that was the most important consideration. I was really nervous and made sure I was at the place she suggested in plenty of time and sat near the door wondering who would come. I'd somehow managed to turn this into a blind date situation from my viewpoint. When she arrived, I recognised her as the lady who had been much older than the others, I think that she was at least ten years older than me. Thankfully, she did most of the talking; all I had to do was listen and ask interested questions and make occasional remarks that showed I was paying attention – she liked talking about herself. A couple of times she said – "and what about you?" Then I'd begin to sketch out some basic biography before she quickly got back onto a much more interesting subject – herself. By the end of the evening

I knew all about her hysterectomy, hip replacement, divorce and mastectomy, as well as plenty of other things in her life that she was unhappy about. She was a smart lady and had worked up to a high level in a company. When I e-mailed her afterwards to say thank you for meeting me, she replied that she didn't think we had much in common and consequently didn't wish to see me again – that was fine by me. The situation made me feel sad because when I'd dated girls as a young man it was different; there was a positive aspect to it, a sense of possibilities. Going on dates when you're young is fun but when you're older it can be a grim experience; the dating landscape doesn't look so wonderful from late middle age. It was a cheerless revelation to see how much things had changed in between the shutdown many years ago and my recent fragile re-awakening. Yet, it was only one date with one lady. There are plenty of other women looking for someone, perhaps there's one somewhere that I could be right for?

The Beginning of Amazement

I can't recall how it came into my possession; perhaps I swapped something for it or won it in a game or challenge of some kind. I think I was about twelve or thirteen. I do remember the effect it had upon me – my first girlie magazine. A complete one, not just a couple of pages torn out from some dog-eared copy, but the whole thing. I was transfixed by its contents, particularly the girl in the centre pages – I thought that she was the most beautiful sight I'd ever seen. I felt a sweet warmth arising inside me when I looked at her pictures, the unknowing early stirrings of sexual desire. She was my first fantasy girl; all I did was cuddle and kiss her in my dreams – I had little idea then what else might be possible. As it turns out, I'm not really capable of much more these days either. Perhaps I've travelled full circle but missed out on the journey.

Counselling

After a wobble, when I felt a strong attraction to a woman and had some dark and despairing thoughts as a result, I decided that I wasn't going to let this happen anymore. I went to see my GP and was referred for counselling. Several months later I saw a therapist for six fifty-minute sessions; by that time I was feeling a lot more positive than when I had been first referred but it seemed like a good idea to try and fix the roof whilst the sun was shining. I learnt some interesting things about the critical self, the dynamic of fear, and how we're all a bit broken one way or another. The counsellor was a big advocate of mindfulness. I bought a book about this, but I've never really incorporated the exercises into my daily life. I think that counselling might have helped a lot when I was younger, nearer the time of my castration, but twenty-three years afterwards was probably too late to make a difference.

Records on the Kitchen Label

Fabulous Nobody – *Love and the City* (7" vinyl)
Trilemma – *Crowded Wilderness* (7" vinyl)
By Coastal Cafe – *At Budokan* (7" vinyl)
The Groove Criminals – *Kicking Up Dust* (7"
   vinyl)
Stars of Aviation – *Snow on Snow* (CD)
Guitare Brothers – *Remix Moi* (7" vinyl)
   Remixes by Bumpy, DJ Ordeal, Transistor 6,
   Waverunner
Riders – *Riders* (7" vinyl)
By Coastal Cafe – *Old Cartoons* (12" vinyl LP)
Horowitz – *Frosty Cat Songs* (12" vinyl LP)
Stars of Aviation – *Marie et L'Accordeon* (7" vinyl)

Unfulfilled

"The imagination of a eunuch dwells more and longer upon the material of love than that of man and woman… supplying, so far as he can, by speculation, the place of pleasures he can no longer enjoy." – John Quincy Adams

Why exactly the sixth president of the United States would be offering an opinion about eunuchs and their frustrated impulses is not clear, but he made an astute observation. Having a great deal of unreleased, and un-releasable, energy building up inside you leads to an increased consideration of what you don't and can never have. I take a deep, but entirely academic, interest in sexual and relationship matters. I voraciously read articles and listen to items that discuss various aspects of these wonders that are lost to me. It's as if knowing dry facts about somewhere I cannot physically experience somehow brings me closer to a sense of being there – like devouring travelogues from impossible destinations in forever distant lands.

Juice

Several types of synthetic testosterone are available, usually in either gel form or injection. Gels are rubbed onto your skin daily; the testosterone is absorbed and enters your bloodstream. Guys using this are warned not to cuddle their girlfriends or partners for a while afterwards until the gel is dry, so that the testosterone cannot be passed on by skin-to-skin contact. It wouldn't be good if your girlfriend began exhibiting male characteristics, would it? You're not to even think about going near a pregnant woman until you're dressed. I disliked gel as it felt like I was performing my daily Eunuch Ritual when I applied it, plus I was impotent when using it. There are several different injections available. For several years I used one that caused me to pile on weight; some people said that it made me aggressive, but more importantly – I could get erections with it. It seems that they stopped making it in this country some years ago because too many side-effects were noted; aggression, mood-swings, obesity and sexual rampancy amongst them. It's used by steroid-abusing bodybuilders to bulk up their muscles, and the dosages that some of them take are quite dangerous. Since I stopped using this injection, I've been impotent.

I have in the past had abnormally high and also negligibly low levels of testosterone and found noticeable differences. When my levels of the hormone have been high, I've felt a tension within my body, a heat coursing through me. I put on weight, but also felt much stronger. Some people suggested I was more aggressive than normal; I was "pumped" and felt rather good that way. When my levels have been low, I've had a more placid outlook and an increased tendency towards sentimentality. I've also had a lot less "get-up-and-go", often feeling a bit indifferent about things generally, and my physical capabilities diminish – I become tired more easily, whilst my memory also seems to become a bit patchy.

It's not as simple a matter as quantity or volume though; hormones in the bloodstream require appropriate receptors to function correctly before they can have any effect. Hormones are a complex matter, with a wide variety of possible individual responses and outcomes.

I'm not certain that testosterone itself is necessarily the primary driver of the male psyche, but it may certainly turbo-charge the engine. The mechanism of masculinity is a construction of learnt attitudes that arise from upbringing and cultural influences. I think that testosterone affects the physical responses to stimuli but that social conditioning is the critical factor that determines most male behaviour.

Sometimes it seemed to me like the accelerator in a car; when my testosterone levels were high, the slightest touch would cause the engine to roar, but when levels were low repeated treading on the pedal would bring little response. What sort of motorist you are doesn't necessarily depend upon the type of vehicle in which you find yourself, but you might change your style of driving accordingly. I am now stuck in an old piece of scrap that has no wheels or engine – I'm going nowhere. It doesn't really matter what fuel is put in the tank.

Making Friends With Myself

For many years, I was in my body but didn't really have a connection with it. Of course, I could register physical sensations, but we didn't have full diplomatic relations with each other. I was neglectful of my physical aspect, perhaps because I was repelled by what I had become. I put on quite a bit of weight after castration, but still played football and cricket. When I later gave up smoking, I bloated up and have never lost the weight I put on. I also stopped participating in sports about this time and have been obese ever since. I didn't respect myself or my body, though I didn't have any inkling at the time that this was the case. I suppose I just didn't care anymore, I felt that I wasn't worth looking after.

After too long, I slowly began to pay attention to what my body was telling me; the messages weren't good. I realised that I must take better care of myself. It took a long time, but I became friendlier with myself and my body. Now I can feel it differently, am more fully aware of what it says, and I listen to what it tells me. When I have had a cup of tea and a piece of cake, I can feel the rush moving around me whereas before I would binge on industrial quantities of sugar and not feel anything much. I'm still fat, and have a long way to go, but I've not completely given up yet either. Slowly, the internal dialogue in my head became more respectful and kind. I even started to address myself by my name, not the hateful terms of abuse that I'd been using for years. Instead of relentlessly bullying and undermining myself I began to be a friend to me. I really needed that.

Samizdat

These were underground publications produced and circulated in the Soviet Union from the 1950s to the late 1980s. An oppressive censorship was enforced by the KGB; the state had full control of printing presses and photocopiers, leaving little room for the expression of ideas that met with official disproval. A form of renegade literature arose, firstly in Moscow and Leningrad, and eventually spread across the various republics that constituted the Soviet Union. The name is a combination of two Russian words and means "self-published". Copies of publications were secretly made and distributed discreetly by hand, often they were produced using carbon paper or were sometimes even handwritten. They reached only a tiny readership, being in possession of such material was dangerous. The content was usually concerned with political issues, often consisting of reports of trials and occurrences that were kept out of the official news, as well as opinion pieces. Sometimes the material dealt with cultural matters or was of a religious or spiritual nature. Some contained sexual content or pornography. Producers of Samizdat were liable to surveillance and persecution by the all-pervading state apparatus; many were arrested and imprisoned, but the form still survived until the glasnost era in the 1980s, when it experienced a resurgence before seeing the collapse of the totalitarian state that had attempted to subjugate and destroy such freedom of expression.

Promises (to an Unknown Lover)

I will –

- hug you (often)
- remove spiders and unscrew tight lids on jars when requested (without comment)
- listen to your stories (and if I've already heard the one you're telling several times before, will pay attention as if it was the first time you've told it to me)
- accept that you love the cat more than you love me (and always will)
- bring you back to earth when you're being just a bit too much (it is anticipated that this will be necessary only on very rare occasions)
- remind you how beautiful you are, particularly when (unbelievably) you think you're not

Haircut

Earinus was a most beautiful young Greek boy, who was sent to Rome as a gift to the Emperor Domitian. He was castrated to prevent him losing his pretty looks and worked as an imperial cupbearer. Several poems were written about him; it appears that he may have been the emperor's favourite and was an unusually wilful slave who came to have much influence over the debauched ruler. The emperor issued decrees to outlaw the castration of young boys for the purpose of producing sex workers – historians suggest that this was at the urging of Earinus. Unusually, he was granted his freedom whilst still a teenager, and in 94 AD committed the unprecedented act of standing up in public and cutting his hair. In Ancient Rome, youths grew their hair long and cut it off along with their first beard upon reaching manhood; a eunuch was expected to have long hair until death. Earinus had no beard, but his defiant gesture may have been a statement that he, one of a particularly despised and marginalised group, was just as good as any man in the empire. Nothing is known of what happened to him afterwards.

Just Looking

Sometimes, I look at a woman and wish I could feel a hot rush of lust for her. I may feast my eyes upon her, but that's all I do. I don't imagine being with her; any fantasies that I consciously summon are barren and disconnected. So, I just look, mesmerised. The more I look at her, the more compelling she becomes, and the more I become painfully aware of what I lack – an exquisite torture. I reluctantly tear my gaze away from her with an agitated sadness, despising my inadequacy.

Sad Realisation

I built a castle to take refuge in – somewhere I could feel safe and protected. Now, I curse myself for becoming a captive in a prison of my own making.

The Shadow of Goodbye

I still think about doing it sometimes. Not so that I might actually go through with it, but when I'm down and despondent, I imagine taking flight from some high ledge. I spread my wings and fly, upwards to the stars – who's to say that I could not? It is only a passing darkness cast by distortions in the sky of my mind; soon, the idea has gone.

Finding What You're Looking For

It is said that we cannot find happiness if we search for it; it is not a destination, but a way of travelling. Sometimes we can become so focused on finding something that it becomes elusive, precisely because we are looking for it so desperately.

After my castration I was determined that I would lead a meaningful and useful life; that though I could only leave a small footprint behind me, I would have a positive effect upon the world and make a contribution to collective human wellbeing. I invested myself heavily in my work in the NHS, and became very involved with the hospital that I worked in. I believed that helping people was a virtuous endeavour, and it was one that absorbed me greatly. Before I had only played sports; now I took on other roles – running teams, organising events, becoming a match and league official. It gave me a vicarious happiness to help bring enjoyment to other people. I had always loved music as a listener but now set up a very small, and financially unsuccessful, record label. Later on, I organised gigs and live music events that were run on a similarly un-business-like basis, but allowed me to enjoy the glow of other people's energy. I contributed to various charities, many that helped children, and was giving 15% of my salary to these each month. At work I became a trade union representative. Though I hadn't ever been any good at speaking up for myself, I became very good at speaking up for others. All these activities seemed very worthy, but they didn't really make me happy in the slightest. They were only distractions that diverted my attention from myself and the gaping emptiness that had opened up inside me and became increasingly painful each day. I sought to *be* a good person, one that *did* good – but this didn't make me *feel* good about who I was, or the life I was leading. I don't think that you can seek to give meaning or purpose to your life by trying to construct these things from extraneous material; they can only become possible if you cultivate an environment that will cause them to grow within you. The best conditions for this occur when you have a healthy relationship with yourself, and a good level of self-knowledge – I possessed neither. The energy that can create happiness arises from inside you, not some external source. You won't ever find what you look for if you search for it, but you can make it happen once you learn to use abilities that we all possess. A pre-occupation with happiness may actually make you less happy, an obsession with a certain idea of love might cause your life to be a loveless one. Perhaps it is the same with purpose and meaning too.

Shame

Each day I am reminded of what I am, and what I'm not. The name is irredeemable; there are some things that it will never be possible to be proud of.

True shame is a deeply personal torment. It is neither guilt nor embarrassment. Guilt is a negative response arising from wrongdoing, whilst embarrassment is more concern about others' reactions when a publicly held standard has not been met.

Shame is a core experience of being that emphasises lack of worth and inadequacy. Shame tells you how useless and bad you are, regularly and often. Whilst those full of guilt may feel an urge to confess, the shameful can only retreat into a secret prison where they condemn themselves to a wretched existence. All beings desire the light however; some may shrink from it, whilst at the same time dreaming of walking in it. The cold darkness is certain and provides a painful re-assurance whilst you destroy yourself slowly. One day it will be too late.

Joke

I am the joke that is never funny, told in unheard whispers; an object of ridicule and contempt. As for pity, I have lavished too much of that upon myself already. I am surrounded by those who are what I am not, and never can be. I feel a vicarious pleasure in others' happiness, but this regularly collapses into short bursts of jealousy and resentment. The world has much beauty; I have learnt to see it all around, yet I am disconnected from it often, isolated within an invisible bubble of my own making.

An illusion of remission is brought by the adoption of cynicism, as if to devalue the world is to increase one's relative worth. This only brings further suffering as you acquire a sour disposition that diminishes your capacity for happiness and your ability to experience being alive.

Updates Are Available

Software is complex; the operating systems of each individual contain many programmes that are in a constant state of flux and re-write themselves continually unnoticed. Long ago, an error was detected somewhere in one of these; it was shut down and quarantined. I have programmed my own unhappiness, a realisation that brings further condemnation upon me, further shame at my inadequacy. Programmes can always be re-installed though. Updates are available.

Unknown Magic

A school orchestra were murdering a light classical staple at the supermarket entrance. As I hurried past, something unexpected caught my ear, causing me to stop. I put my bags down and listened, allowing the music to wash over me and fill me up inside. When the piece finished, I applauded enthusiastically; a passer-by might have taken me for a commendably supportive parent.

Teamwork requires that each individual must be aware of their role in the bigger plan and conform to this. Solo performance allows for unscheduled excursions, where liberties might discreetly be taken, and possibilities explored. When performing as part of a collective, each player must reign in individual tendencies and hold their position within the formation, otherwise mayhem might ensue. Apart from end-of-term concerts, this was probably the only time some of the members of this orchestra were ever going to play in public; perhaps a lot of them knew it too. This gave licence to reckless abandonment; instead of playing within themselves, many took this opportunity to slip off such inhibition and their own technical limitations and go beyond anywhere they had been before. They had pushed far past the boundaries of their capabilities into a place where normal rules no longer apply, an unmappable region where magic is made. Order had been dismantled; a new equilibrium of chaos had been arrived at by chance.

Here was a crowd of solo performers who regarded the given score as a suggested place of departure, not a destination. They were stretching in different directions, pulling the music apart; and by doing so, transforming it into something new, misshapen, and unspeakably beautiful.

One grey day, in a drab little place, the greatest orchestra in the history of the world played – and nobody knew.

Escort Girls

The only women I have cuddled in over twenty years are ones that I have paid to be with. Why would an impotent eunuch visit an escort girl? Perhaps it's because I'm an inadequate freak, who is distorted psychologically and emotionally. I felt that the only way I could feel a woman's skin against mine was to pay for this privilege. It seemed to me that I was never going to have a relationship for the rest of my days; I was worthless as a man and this was the best that I could hope for. I still occasionally think about doing this once more when feeling particularly tormented. It was always an unsatisfactory experience, the only rational reason to visit these ladies is to fuck them – and I'm incapable of that. When I was in my darkest place, the illusion of physical intimacy was a hollow consolation that I sought in an effort to distract me from my wretchedness. When you've not been touched for a long time, the prospect of feeling the body of a woman against yours can seem very appealing. For the most part, I found the ladies to be pleasant, smart and interesting people. I fully understand that any charm they displayed towards me was completely fake; it's an entirely transactional situation as far as they're concerned. In such an impersonal scenario I knew that the girl couldn't care less about me, that she would forget about me as soon as I'd walked out of the door afterwards. This made it easier in one way, whilst also making it even more pointless in another. It seemed to provide a small solace to caress and hold an attractive young woman in my arms. This was a distraction that I sought when my perspective was distorted, it seemed to briefly soothe my suffering a little. I would really want an emotional connection with any woman that I was with, that's something that you can't buy. Perhaps it is something that I will never have, and sometimes, in weaker and more self-indulgent moments, that thought makes me wonder if life is really worth living.

Creep

Many people will find the idea of a fat old eunuch having unfulfillable sexual thoughts and romantic feelings about women to be a skin-crawlingly creepy idea.

I'm not afraid of anyone's contempt though; you cannot despise me any more than I have myself for many years. So, please don't waste any of your disdain upon me – I am unworthy of your scorn. I'm a neutered freak, my kind have revolted normal people for thousands of years. Of course I'm a creep, what else would I be?

Buying Books

I buy books a lot faster than I read them; I've got quite a few at home that I haven't got around to starting yet. Perhaps acquiring a book is a statement of intent in itself, a signpost to an unvisited horizon that you hope to travel towards someday. Purchasing one is an aspirational gesture that isn't always consummated by reading.

Golden Gate Bridge Survivors

The span across the San Francisco Bay is a famous landmark; it's also a prolific suicide location. Anything between 1,500 and 1,700 people are thought to have leapt from the bridge; perhaps as many as thirty of these have survived, some with serious internal injuries and severe fractures. One thing that has been consistently mentioned by those survivors who have spoken about their experience is that as they began their plunge towards destruction, the powerful realisation overwhelmed them that they actually wanted to *live*! Even though they'd given the matter lengthy consideration beforehand, once they'd committed themselves to ending their lives, they knew that this was something they didn't really want at all.

What Are the Odds?

There is a class of men that women describe as being "single for a reason" – I suspect that I may just qualify for this category, apart from not *actually* being a man. I've got more issues than *Vogue*, and more hang-ups than the Tate. My dating pool is the equivalent of a dried-up watering hole in the Serengeti during a particularly severe drought.

The In-Call

You look at the website, check the rota to see who's available. You call the number, questions and answers are exchanged; a booking is made. The lady on the 'phone is usually good at matching up girls' skill sets to the client's requirements. An address is texted to you, an apartment block. You arrive in the neighbourhood beforehand. You wait until it's time, then you let them know you're there. An apartment number is texted to you. You press the buzzer; an intercom voice tells you to come up. You take the lift, or climb the stairs, then find the correct corridor – the corridors all look the same. You notice that your heart is thumping; you take a couple of deep breaths. You find the door, double-checking on your 'phone that it's the right number. You knock – not too loud. You hear heels on the other side; sometimes she looks through the spyglass for a second or two to check. Then the latch clicks, and the door opens a little. She looks good, they always do. She smiles, her head angled slightly, causing her hair to slip off her shoulder. She knows your name; she's been waiting for you. She opens the door wider and invites you in.

She asks you to sit down; sometimes she'll ask you if you want a drink. Water – your mouth's dry. There is small talk, preliminaries approached. Some agencies have a policy; you must have a shower first. Most leave it to the girl's discretion. You've spruced up anyway – like you're actually going on a date or something. They're very smart, observant. They have to be; doing that work. You hand her the money, she takes it and goes to put it somewhere safe, after checking the amount is correct. She has to call the agency too, let them know it's going ahead. She'll call them later as well, to let them know you've left, afterwards.

Covers

A song belongs to whoever is singing it; copyright ownership is just a legal technicality. Often "original" songs are anything but original, just recycled sameness, whilst some singers and artists perform cover versions that have so much creativity invested in them that an old song becomes new, played for the first time ever. Songs can also belong to whoever hears them, an audience can listen in vastly different ways. That's part of why music can be so magical, nobody owns it really.

Little Balls

Even when I had balls, they were defective ones. It turned out that both of mine were abnormal; maybe this accounts for me having been a shy boy who lacked confidence and was a bit too sensitive. When I had a CT scan, after having my first testicle removed, the report stated that my remaining testicle was small. It was exactly the same size as they'd both been during my life up until then. So maybe there *is* something to having big balls and being a real man.

The Best Part

When I visited escorts, I didn't really know what I actually wanted to do with them once I was with them. I was impotent, and did not feel desire for them, but acknowledged that a sublimated sexual impulse had led to my visiting them. Loneliness was a big factor too, as well as a deformed sense of identity. I can't honestly say that I gained any pleasure from being with them, but I felt calmer afterwards – as though an emotional bubble had been deflated. I enjoyed running my hands over the smooth skin of a woman, but it was as if I wasn't there and it all wasn't real somehow. The part that I really liked was when we just lay quietly together, saying nothing, our bodies wrapped in a silent embrace. A few girls aren't so keen on doing this, but most don't mind at all; some mentioned that they felt sleepy when I cuddled them like this. Once, one girl actually dropped off. She was cross with herself when she awoke, you can't let your guard down in her kind of work. For a few moments when I held a girl like that, and she lay in my arms, I felt as though I was taking care of her. For a fleeting instant, I almost felt like I was a man again.

Timid

Many times, in past years, I would find myself attracted to a lady who seemed nice, but if I spoke with her, I would be very cautious about showing any interest in her. I lacked confidence and compiled a long list of reasons in my head why a woman wouldn't ever want me – I expected to fail and therefore I did. Perhaps I only made lame attempts at approaching ladies because deep down I didn't feel that I deserved a woman, as I wasn't really a man.

Very occasionally, *really* occasionally, a lady would show a tentative interest in me, but I would respond like a sea anemone withdrawing its tentacles at the approach of potential danger. I feared the humiliation and contempt that might follow if she discovered my shameful secret.

Locks on a Canal

Where the Rochdale Canal passes under Oxford Road there is a small set of railings. These bear nearly six hundred padlocks with paired initials upon them – declarations of love. I always smile when I pass there. There are few other places in the city that would be suitable for such a collection. Once a couple of similar padlocks appeared on the curved bridge just north of Piccadilly Basin, but were soon removed.

Superstar

I visited a lady who was regarded by some as being the best escort in Manchester. She was very pretty and intelligent, and apparently fluent in many languages. I heard that one European client had seen her when he was in town on business and had since been flying in regularly at weekends just so he could be with her again. She had lots of charm and knew how to use it; you couldn't help falling under her spell. If international peace or trade talks ever get deadlocked anywhere, they should call her in – with her charisma even the most intransigent leaders would be best friends in no time. I told her not to bother attempting to turn me on, as it would be a waste of time. She still tried but soon conceded defeat; she said that such a thing had never happened to her before. I just held her in my arms whilst we talked, exchanging stories and book recommendations.

Lost on the Yellow Brick Road

A strange little group is wandering lost within the city of Munchkinchester. They are all looking for something, but don't know where to find it. The cowardly lion seeks courage so that he might become brave. The stupid scarecrow seeks a brain so that he might gain wisdom. The tinman wants a heart so that he may be able to love…and the eunuch wishes to have the balls to be a man. Dorothy went home but didn't know where that place really was – none of us do. The Wizard is proving elusive; maybe he doesn't really live here, perhaps he's an illusion. The Good Witch of the North has left a message – "You've always had the power my dear, you just had to learn it for yourself." What did she mean by that?

Is it all a dream? Are these characters only creations of a warped imagination, my imagination? They are all me, and I am them. Oh dear, perhaps there isn't going to be a happy ending.

Ones That Got Away

Yukio Shige was away from the cliffs when one of his volunteer team spotted a girl standing near the edge. The girl told the volunteer to say nothing, so the volunteer just stood with her in silence for a long while, then gently initiated a dialogue that lasted for over an hour. A couple of police officers turned up and got involved; one of them meant well but said the wrong thing. The officer asked the girl to consider how worried her parents must be – the girl said "Sayonara" and leapt.

Don Ritchie was talking to a young man at Sydney Gap who stared straight ahead at the sea. After a while, Don thought that he was getting somewhere and asked the young man if he'd like to come to his house across the road for a beer. The young man said – "No" and stepped forward. The wind blew his hat off as he went over the edge, Don instinctively caught it and was left standing alone holding the young man's hat in his hand.

Kevin Briggs leant upon the rail talking to a man who was standing on the ledge of the Golden Gate Bridge. The man asked if he was familiar with the story of Pandora's Box. Kevin said that he was; the man responded that sometimes there was no hope left in the bottom of the box. He then jumped.

Chen Si had an elderly relative who had become unable to look after himself; the old man's family argued over who should care for him, nobody wanted to do it. He heard their discussions and killed himself rather than be an unwanted burden.

My Greatest Foe

Me. I am my most terrible enemy, the one that has brought devastation upon my own life. I knew the weaknesses to be hammered at, the flaws to be exploited. I made a good job of messing myself up. Please make sure that you are not your own worst enemy; be friends with yourself if possible.

Free

It took a long time for the neural pathways that had been scorched into my brain to become dormant. I feel happier now that I have liberated myself from a damaging habit. Once I had encountered pornography and begun using it regularly, my libido became deformed and inflamed, as if on psychological steroids. Gradually I have healed and returned to a more natural form of being. I am saddened that I was oppressed by malign spirits in my head, but proud that I have banished them after much struggle.

NQ Kaleidoscope

I remember the Northern Quarter before it had this title bestowed upon it. Back then it was a dark place, full of decay, and with a slightly forbidding vibe.

In winter afternoons, the sun shines straight along Oldham Street. When it has been raining or snowing, the road glistens with a blinding light. The street is truly paved with gold on such days.

Often pallets are left on Spear Street, opposite the back entrance of Night & Day; some are brand new and might make good recycled furniture that would look great in your place.

You may notice metal kerbs; apparently Manchester's one of the last cities that still has them. They were used because the wheels of heavy carts used to crack stone kerbs.

They say that there's a hidden Banksy on the electricity sub-station situated on Tib Lane. When the council realised that he'd left a work there it was shielded behind a protective plastic cover. Gradually, posters were stuck upon this and now it's blanketed with them. We could go and see it, stand there and wonder what it looks like – a concealed installation, a secret unrevealed.

Several summers ago, a lady sat on a folding chair behind a small folding desk on the pavement on Thomas Street. She had a typewriter and a sign – custom erotica. She did a fair bit of trade; the keys clicked-clacked behind her brain as she composed pieces for all shades of love and desire.

There's plenty of street art to see. A while back green mushrooms with very long, thin stalks appeared on walls here and there. We can walk around and see what's new; Spear Street and Warwick Street usually have something good.

Double Hibakusha

Hibakusha is the name given to those directly involved in the nuclear bombings of Hiroshima and Nagasaki – it translates as "explosion-affected person". It is known that at least 69 individuals were unfortunate enough to have been present at both targets, but only one of these sought official recognition for this from the Japanese government. Tsutomu Yamaguchi was preparing to leave Hiroshima when he saw a plane fly overhead and drop something. He was knocked over by the blast, his eardrums were ruptured and much of his body was covered in burns. The next day he returned to his hometown – Nagasaki. After being treated for his injuries he reported for work at the Mitsubishi Corporation and was in the process of explaining to a sceptical supervisor what had happened a few days before in Hiroshima when another blinding flash in the sky was followed once more by a devastating blast and a shower of radioactive black rain.

Towards the end of his life Tsutomu Yamaguchi became an outspoken supporter for nuclear disarmament and the abolition of such weapons. He sought official recognition of his double hibakusha status to publicise his views.

Unisex Hormones

Whilst women have testosterone as part of their natural hormonal make up, it is also the case the oestrogen is part of the male constitution. Both sexes share the classically "male" and "female" hormones, but in varying proportions. It's a complex matter that is not as simple as gender stereotyping might suggest. There are several other factors that account for a wide range of individual variations, such as proteins in the blood and different hormone receptors in various organs. There has been little research on the subject but there are suggestions that oestrogen influences male sexual and reproductive function. One study, conducted on rats, found that males with higher oestrogen levels displayed an increased tendency to aggressive behaviour. Maybe hormones and their effects upon men and women isn't as black and white a matter as we might assume.

Hidden Codes

The universe does not follow any plan and is not compelled to conform to any formulae. Infinite randomness is the purest and most perfect order. Patterns may be discerned in the movements of everything if there is a desire to see such things.

The operating software of consciousness creates and

updates itself continuously. It manifests in the pro-grammes that arise from infinite interactions with itself. Its countless articulations alter each other eternally, causing shifts within itself that lead to a perfect stillness. Everything is conjured from nothing; both are the same.

And you, a seemingly insignificant aspect of irrel-evance, contain all the codes within you that might explain and make sense of it all – and you don't realise it. You have no idea of your vast importance.

Creative

There is a saying – be creative or die. Once you stop being creative in some way, you shrivel inside and will remain that way until you begin trying to make some-thing beautiful once more. You don't have to be an "artist" who expresses themselves in painting or music; talent is nice to have but is not necessary. With some people it's cooking, or gardening, or home decoration. It might be your clothes and hair, how you make a bed, the way you write a letter. The light may rise up within you when you dance in your room when no-one is watching you, when you wrap someone's present, or set out the table. The smallest actions might be an instrument upon which you may play, the world is enriched by such tiny acts of love. This is true art, an unconscious attempt to express that which is beyond expression.

A Train to Nowhere

I desperately look out of the window; this isn't the journey I intended to make. Can we go back please? No, that's impossible. I missed changes because I wasn't paying attention; perhaps I'd nodded off or was reading some tedious book when we stopped at stations long past and impossible to return to. What am I going to do now? I'm trapped. The carriage speeds along the track, taking me further away from places that I had once hoped to go to. I only had one ticket, and I wasted it.

Sorry

I used to apologise all the time; for speaking, for taking up space, for being what I am. People noticed this and commented upon it a lot. Somehow, whilst compiling this banal jigsaw, I began to stop constantly saying sorry to people. I realised that I'd lived my life to please other people, had subordinated myself to the approval of others. Too late have I understood this and wish that I had lived my life for myself instead. I think that it would have been a much happier one if I had done so.

Blame

I don't blame anyone except myself for having had, in many regards, an unfulfilled life. I lacked the character to deal with the situation that confronted me and didn't have the awareness and knowledge to be able to respond to my trivial challenges in the best way. I wish that I had understood the importance of self-knowledge twenty years ago; I would have led a much different life. I shut down and shrivelled when I should have stood up and challenged my emotions. You have to fight for happiness. I allowed myself to be overcome with a whiny self-pity, and a destructive self-hatred; I contained all these poisons secretly within myself and suffered the consequences.

Wisdom

Socrates stated that the unexamined life is not worth living. The suggestion seems to be that self-knowledge is vital to having a fulfilled life, and that existing in a state of ignorance is to spurn true happiness. Burying your head in the sand, or ignoring uncomfortable ideas, is a harmful strategy to adopt. The problem is that sometimes you might *think* you know who you are, and why you perceive the world as you do, but how do you know that your understanding is a true one? You don't usually know that you're making a mistake whilst committing it, it's only later that your error might become apparent and wisdom arise. Even then, learning the wrong lessons will lead us even further away from the prospect of living a meaningful and happy life. Perhaps a poor examination is more harmful than no examination? I wonder what Socrates would have had to say about that.

As a young man, I constantly examined my actions and the reasons for them in a continuous attempt to be a better person. I placed myself under a critical surveillance that inevitably found me wanting; I was never good enough for my conscience. After many years blundering in psychological twilight, I have come to realise that any true examination must be done in circumstances of kindness and acceptance, not prejudice and contempt. A poor examination of yourself and your life will cause you to remain in the darkness of ignorance. The light comes from love, and it must begin within you, for you yourself, before it can shine for anyone else. Socrates also suggested that the unlived life wasn't worth examining, a proposition that crushes me every time I consider it.

Grief

It is sometimes suggested that the bereaved cannot love again until they have resolved their grief. It took too many years before I realised that this might apply to me; I didn't even know that I was experiencing a kind of grief. Perhaps I needed to mourn what I had lost, but I wouldn't accept that I had anything to feel bad about; there were many people with bigger problems than mine, I could've been a lot worse off. Whilst that may have been true it was no reason to pretend that something doesn't need fixing if it badly requires repair. It is negligent to ignore obvious problems. I wasted a large portion of my life with a retarded, shut-down outlook. There are things I might have been, and things I could have done, had I known how to be a better version of me.

How do you grieve for a person that never was, and the loves unloved? It seems a bit too self-absorbed, it's much easier just to dismiss such ideas and not deal with them. It might be simpler to ignore uncomfortable feelings that don't conform to a simplified idea of how things are supposed to be, but this will likely lead to bigger trouble in the long run. Resisting difficult feelings only makes them greater and more challenging to deal with later, because you are going to have to face up to them eventually one way or another.

I have heard many people describing their grief. The emptiness, the loss of meaning, the aching engagement in pursuits once shared with their loved one, the attempts to fill the time with "interests" that have little real interest. I powerfully recognise the feelings expressed, but never got to experience the happiness that's ending caused such great pain. If grief is the price of love, then I've overpaid several times over for something that I never had.

I did not lose a loved one, I lost intangible possibilities, and then I lost myself. It was me that caused this to occur because I did not act in my best interests, I felt I had to conform to an unrealistic ideal. I did not grieve, I considered that it would be undignified and self-indulgent. I did not know myself and did not know how to deal with difficult feelings.

Lost in the Desert

I have learnt the ways of the wilderness so well. What may seem barren to the passing visitor, actually contains obscure subtleties that slowly reveal themselves. I belong in this harsh emptiness now; it has become my home. I still retain vague recollections of another place but doubt that I would be able to adjust if I were to return there. The heat burns the air and distorts dreams into shimmering holograms; I sit on a rock and watch them dance in front of me. I have become well adapted to this savage environment, and wander further into uncharted territories, daring them to destroy me once and for all. I desire my own annihilation but am constantly surprised at my ability to survive in the wasteland.

The Last Eunuch of China

Sun Yaoting was castrated by his father as a child and went on to serve the last Emperor. The communists took control in 1949 and despised the castrated freaks who were weird relics of the hated feudal system which they'd overthrown. He was lucky to survive the Cultural Revolution in the 1960s; his family were fearful of any connection with the old ways being discovered and destroyed his "treasure" – his preserved genitals. These were buried with eunuchs so that they might be a complete man in death that they hadn't been in life, therefore giving them a chance of being a man in the next life. Sun lived long enough to acquire some celebrity status as a witness to the last days of imperial China before passing away in 1996.

Life Lessons

Bronnie Ware was an Australian palliative care nurse who looked after patients with terminal cancer in the last days of their lives. She would talk with them and listen to their stories. She noted that as they approached the end, they each found peace. She also realised that they consistently expressed the same five regrets about their lives, and later wrote a book about this.

The five regrets of the dying are –

1. I wish I'd had the courage to live a life true to myself, not the life others expected of me
2. I wish I hadn't spent so much time working
3. I wish I'd had the courage to express my feelings
4. I wish I had stayed in touch with my friends
5. I wish that I had let myself be happier

Glimmers

Sometimes, I imagine a woman lying beside me in bed at night, looking out of the window whilst I drive the car, or strolling with me as I walk somewhere. She appears fleetingly, without warning. Occasionally, I fantasise about opening the front door and seeing the lights already on, hearing the sounds of a shared home, feeling the warmth that a woman can bring to a place. These are flickering projections from a parallel universe that is very different from this one, carried here on interstellar breezes; detectable only by lost and distorted souls.

The Ultimate Software

We obsess about the hardware of our lives, but it isn't really so important; it's the software that makes everything happen. God is a name that some give to the essential software of the universal operating system, the computer cloud of all consciousness – the love that is the perfect everything.

Coming Out

My coming out has been rather a drawn-out process. I submitted an exhibit to The Lost & Found exhibition at The Wonder Inn four years ago, which consisted of a prosthetic testicle and a piece of writing relating to loss and discovery. A couple of years later, I had an item published in *The Guardian*'s 'My Life in Sex' series, and now I tell you my story in this unsung love song. I wanted to explain who I was and what I had experienced. Whether people are interested is a different matter; there's no particular reason why anyone would want to know anything about me and my pathetic little life. In addition to indifference, my tale might disgust and offend people too. After the *Guardian* piece was published, some people shunned me. I admit that this hurt me initially, as I wanted to be accepted by them, but I understood their feelings towards me and didn't hold it against them. I was proud that I wasn't scared of disapproval anymore, that I was now strong enough to bear reproach and dislike. Perhaps I will always make some people's flesh crawl because of what I am. Whilst this makes me sad, I'm not going to beat myself up about it.

Ancient Humour

The oldest surviving collection of jokes is the *Philogelos*, a Greek book from the fourth or fifth century AD. Gag number 114 is a joke about a eunuch who doesn't have the balls to have children, but the punchline is missing – appropriately.

Wonderful Things

…the breeze on your face…sunlight…crying when you remember two people who really loved each other…a small gig by an unknown and amazing artist…a really cool girl effortlessly carrying off an awesome look…an unexpected smile from a stranger…a book that you try to read slowly because it is so good that you want it to last as long as possible…a pot of really special loose leaf tea…someone speaking with a delightful voice that caresses your ear…dandelions and buttercups…you… yes, most definitely you…

To Whom It May Concern

To those that mocked and humiliated me: I forgive you completely and unconditionally. I bear you no ill will. You hurt me but I am not angry at you, neither do I pity you or wish to diminish you in any way. I hope that you will be happy, will learn and grow and spread kindness as you pass through this world.

Desert Fish

The West African Lungfish swims in lakes and rivers that lie within a region that regularly experiences a dry season. When water levels begin to fall, they burrow down into the mud, secrete themselves in protective saliva, and their bodies slow down. They breathe and wait beneath dried up, empty water beds. When the rains come with the wet season they return to the newly replenished streams and marshes and live once more.

Hidden Music

It's raining. Can you hear the sound between the drops? Close your eyes and listen; there's something there.

Damp Paper

I sit on the bench reading my book. Wet spots appear on the page, silently at first, then pitter-patter very softly. Drops become bigger and more frequent. People hurry past beneath umbrellas, one or two glances disbelievingly in my direction. The sky is dark when I look up, dark and heavy, but all beneath is shining silver. The book becomes so dazzlingly bright that I can no longer see the words; a glow lights up the pages and blinds me with a realisation that causes my heart to burst all over again. Meanwhile the ancient rain falls from the sky, as it has always done, and as it will continue doing long after I've gone.

A Parting Promise

I would like you to promise me something, please. I very much wish that you will have a better life than I did, that you will not allow yourself to be a loser as I was. You deserve better than that. I hope that I have shown you what *not* to do, and that you have learnt something from this sad, old eunuch. Promise me that you will not waste the opportunities for happiness that this world offers. I hope that you will live your life with a quiet courage and a kind heart, and that you will succeed where I failed. Most of all I hope that you will love as I did not – more than anything I would like that. Thank you for having been here, I'm really glad that you kept me company for a little while. Please take good care of yourself. Goodbye.

The Map Room

Daily expeditions were undertaken; aimlessness, the purpose. He was a reclusive explorer with an anonymous walk-on part in the big production. The surveyor's tools included a camera, wrinkled notebooks and fumbled pens, an arcane disposition. Leatherback turtles travel vast distances of ocean at the speed of a mile an hour and the city has much to tell those that listen and learn its obscure dialects. Fragments of conversation, banal snapshots and humdrum observations may become incongruously profound in another language. He had stumbled painfully, once, but gained an awkward perspective from the fall; his distorted perception allowed him to see the pixels of consciousness. Life is a virtual reality experience, running on haphazard software of perfect insignificance. He saw the unobservable revealed in fleeting conjunctions, astounding secrets hidden in plain view.

He seemed nice enough; friendly and gentle when you got to know him, but he preferred to keep himself to himself for the most part. We hadn't seen him around for a while, prompting a rare visit to his place where an unlocked door was discovered, leading to a revelation – but no explorer. Where did he go? It's an unremarkable place inside, sparse and plain, apart from the notes. A vast collection that must have taken years to accumulate; the observations and measurements from rambling urban excursions attached carefully to the walls of this room, covering them in an expanse of patiently accumulated stories composed of the smallest and most insignificant material. More are scattered across the floor, and a few later ones perhaps, spread upon a table. He has created a map of the city unlike any other.

Small scraps with single sentences, rumpled sheets bearing paragraphs, full pages of composed chapters. A scrambled library of scribbles and print, mosaics of paper and ink that create pictures from words in variable script – some, considered precision; others, breathless improvisation. Allow your eyes to see without looking, randomness creates its own order. Once you've adjusted to its rhythms the room appears to shift with light and shadow, sweeping you up with it in a dance of heart-breaking joy.

Lastly, found upon the table with specific instructions emphasising its importance, a small envelope, only to be opened by one particular person. Look, your name is written upon it, along with this time and place. Of all those in this crowded city, it is to you that the most elusive and precious wisdom is to be given. You open the envelope; there is a folded sheet of paper inside. You read it, but at first it makes no sense at all. Then, the words start moving on the paper; they are dancing for you. Suddenly you see it.

You press the message to your chest and notice that your feet are leading you to the door. Outside the breeze caresses your face, the city is singing, you close your eyes and listen. When you open them again, the lights shimmer below as you glide effortlessly over the beautiful madness. You smile and are overwhelmed by love.